WEIGHT LOSS SUCCESS.

CAN BE YOURS...

John Shaw.

CONTENTS

DISCLAIMER.

This information is not presented by a medical
practitioner and is for educational and informational
purposes only. The content is not intended to be a
substitute for professional medical advice, diagnosis, or
treatment. Always seek the advice of your physician or
other qualified health care provider with any questions
you may have regarding a medical condition. Never
disregard professional medical advice or delay in seeking
it because of something you have read.

Since natural and/or dietary supplements are not FDA
approved they must be accompanied by a two-part
disclaimer on the product label: that the statement has not
been evaluated by FDA and that the product is not
intended to "diagnose, treat, cure or prevent any disease."

YOUR WEIGHT LOSS.

It seems these days that almost everyone has a weight issue, some want to lose weight, some want to gain weight while others just want to maintain the weight they've got without having to resort to a weight loss program that involves excessive exercise or a strict diet.

In fact terms like weight loss, diet plans, how to lose weight, how to lose weight fast, diet, lose weight and how to lose belly fat are amongst the most searched terms on Google and most other search engines.

If you consider, as many people do, that your body is like some kind of engine then you must consider that your body will perform better for longer if it is given the right fuel.

In the [sometimes dim and distant] past there was little or no need for weight loss programs, the only foods that were readily available were those you grew, gathered or caught yourself.

There were no processed foods, no packaged meat, no fruit and vegetables that had been placed into a cold store for weeks or months before they got to your table.

You went into your garden and picked the vegetables you wanted for the day; you went fishing or hunting for your meat.

These activities did two things, not only did they provide good fresh, healthy, nutritious food for you and your family to eat but they also gave you the exercise you needed to maintain a healthy body and a healthy weight.

These days more and more families see both the husband and wife working outside the home and so the whole dynamic of healthy eating, exercise and nutrition has changed.

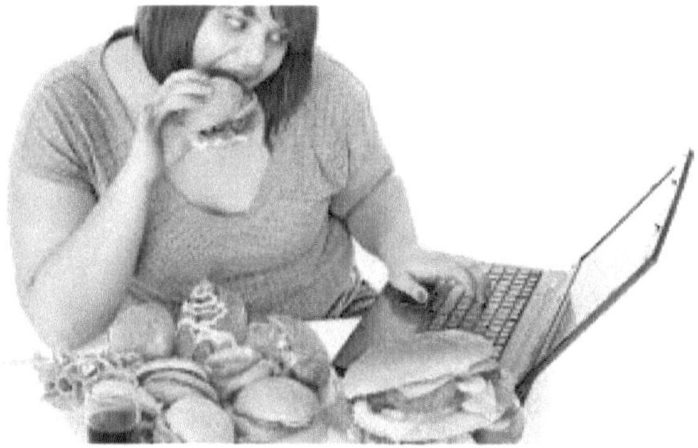

Fast foods have become an accepted "staple" in many people's lives, taking the kids to MacDonalds at the end of a busy day has almost became the norm and let's face it, after a hard day at the office or on the tools who wants to go home and cook?

Even if you do eat at home, these days the average home cooked meal is so laden with artificial preservatives, saturated fats and the like that our bodies are starving for the ingredients that they need and overflowing with the ingredients that they don't need.

Because we don't cook the healthy recipes of our ancestors our bodies aren't getting the nutrition they need our brain tells us that we must put more in, increase the amount of "good stuff" but without considering that with some of that "good stuff" comes a whole truckload of food that really is not good for us at all.

Often our weight loss problem lies right there.

In order for our bodies to get all the nutrition it needs we have to consume much more in total than we otherwise would if our food was fresh and additive free.

To exaggerate, if our food is, for example, fifty percent nutritious and fifty percent "filler" then we have to consume twice as much as if we were getting one hundred percent nutritious food.

This imbalance in our food intake doesn't constitute a healthy diet and results in any number of "problems" with our health.

Weight problems [both too much and also too little weight], skin problems, tiredness, disease, and overall poor health are often the result and although this problem has reached epidemic proportions, we can reverse the effects of poor diet in our own lives if we truly want to.

"Garbage In - Garbage Out."

While this phrase may have been coined for the computer industry, it's very relevant when it comes to our own body.

Every moment that we are alive, our body is busy manufacturing the chemicals, fluids, proteins, and tissues that are required to keep us healthy.

Food, or rather the nutrition that is derived from food, is what the body depends upon to handle all of these tasks.

Everything we eat is used, stored, or discarded by the body.

The body's particular dietary needs can vary widely depending upon what's going on inside and outside of us at any particular time.

Our body makes decisions on what to burn and in what order based upon our pressing energy needs, how long it has been since we last ate and the general condition of our health.

The body burns fuel in a very specific order.

Alcohol is burned first because our bodies have no way to store it for later use, protein is burned next, then carbohydrates and finally fat.

Because fat is consumed last, and the average person has a diet which is rich in fat, our bodies store the fat away to be used at a future time.

How is this fat stored?

You guessed it; it's stored as fatty tissue and that's why we call being overweight "fat".

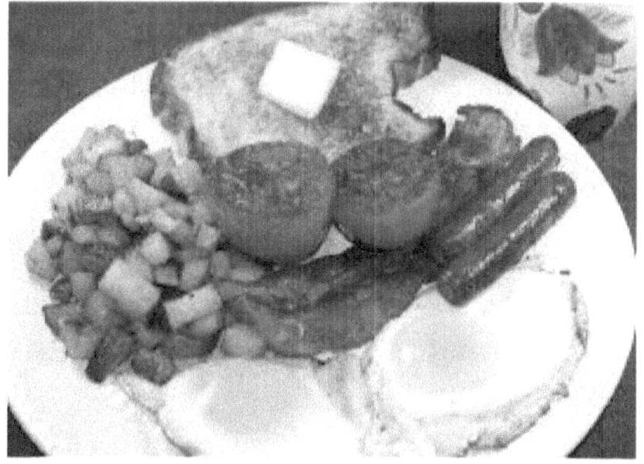

All of this overabundance of fat which is stored in our bodies not only affects our appearance but also has a significant effect on our overall health.

Many studies have proved that excess fat in our diets is directly linked to these medical conditions:

Increased risk of developing certain cancers.

Increased risk of arterial and heart disease due to elevated cholesterol levels.

Increased risk of stroke.

Increased risk of diabetes.

Increased risk of liver disease

and it has a direct impact on the body's immune system.

It is just plain common sense for us to avoid these unnecessary health risks by reducing the amount of fat that we consume every day.

And it's no comfort to know that you're not the only one struggling to lose weight.

Despite the claims that are made almost daily through the media and other sources, there are no wonder diet plans that will work for everyone, no magic diet pills or easy solution to weight loss or weight control in general.

If you want really, really quick weight loss you'll have remove a limb, cut off a leg with a chain saw or perhaps just not eat at all for a week or two, that will work but it's a bit extreme!

While no weight loss program works for everybody, there is something that will give you weight loss success, the challenge is to find it, identify it, and stick to it.

Appetite control works but for some people controlling their appetite may be extremely difficult.

Other weight loss programs try to address the problem by exploring the emotional issues behind our choice of foods (these are the total lifestyle body makeovers, whose techniques include keeping a food journal and coming to terms with one's body image).

Others address the problem by introducing or removing certain foods in your diet plan that are said to either trigger or suppress the appetite.

Still others, like diet pills, act as appetite suppressants.

Other programs rely on nutritional substitutes, like heavy shakes that make you feel full and provide adequate vitamins and minerals, while reducing calories.

For others, it's not appetite that's problematic; it's the kind of food they eat.

Certain diet programs give very strict diet regimens that promote weight loss, because of the way the body digests the food.

Some are short-term, designed to help us shed the kilos over a limited period of time; others suggest long-term lifestyle changes.

The success of these diet programs depend largely on the person's weight loss goals and level of commitment.

Needless to say, if you just want to look good for a certain special event you may not be ready to change your lifestyle completely but if you have health problems and need to control cholesterol levels for example, then a short-term solution would not be very effective.

Other weight loss programs are closely tied with exercise routines.

Of course, not all exercise programs will appeal to everyone; perhaps you might find a visit to the gym appealing or maybe you would prefer something like belly dancing.

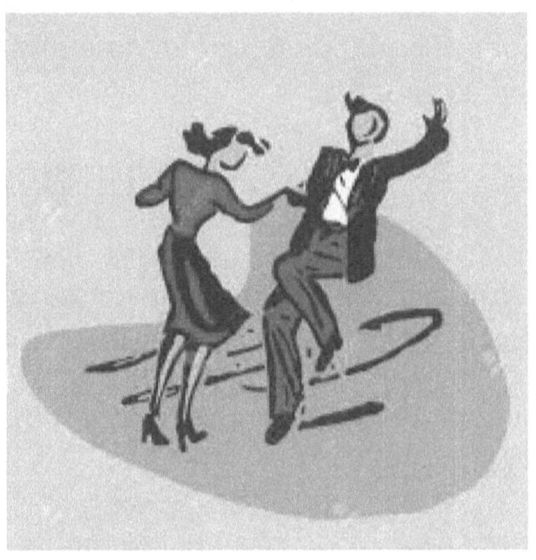

The idea is that you pick what is most interesting to you - the more fun and enjoyment you derive from a routine, the more likely you will stick to it.

The mistake that many people make is that they don't consider what appeals to them when they try a diet or exercise program; they follow what everyone else is doing or jump on the weight loss bandwagon on the mistaken idea that it worked for so-and-so therefore it should work for me.

While it's okay to experiment with different regimens (wouldn't hurt to try anything once), ultimately it is a search to find a weight loss program that is personally appealing.

Another secret to sticking to a diet or exercise program is to have very clear and reasonable goals.

"Be thin" is too general to be meaningful; pinpoint a number, and a date: "Lose 15 pounds by September," and to avoid discouragement, that goal must be humanly achievable and should never compromise with your health.

If a diet makes you dizzy, or radically affects your ability to be fully alert and functional, then stop immediately.

Luckily there is a wide variety of weight loss regimens, there's bound to be one that will help you meet your goals and match your lifestyle.

THE PSYCHOLOGY OF WEIGHT LOSS.

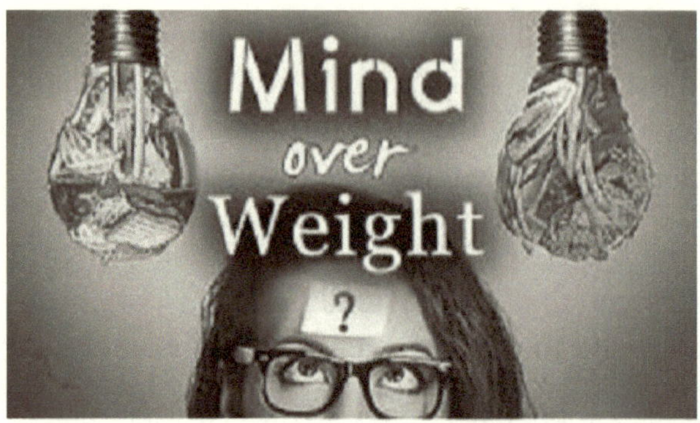

When you see the almost anorexic models on the covers of magazines or you watch your favourite actors and actresses go from year to year without gaining a pound in weight do you ever wonder how it is that they can stay so trim, taut and incredibly slim and you can't?

It may come as a surprise to you to learn that many of those people at some time or another have had difficulty maintaining a healthy weight.

But they were able to overcome their weight problems thanks to a different and somewhat improved view of healthy eating.

You probably don't realize it, but there is a certain psychology at work in successful weight loss.

It is no surprise, then, that the magazine Psychology Today has explored the issue in-depth.

In October of 2004 Psychology Today posted an article on its website detailing the experiences of Diane Berry, a nurse practitioner who studied women who had shed at least 15 pounds and had maintained their weight loss for an average of seven years.

The women shared some important things in common.

One of those things, which turns out to be very important in anyone's quest to lose weight, is that they all had in place a stable support network, many of them had joined Weight Watchers or Jenny Craig or some similar organisation.

Their regular meetings were not only a positive motivating factor but also made them realize that they weren't the only ones struggling with their efforts to lose weight.

These women were also quite unusual in that their weight loss was permanent because the great majority of individuals who lose weight end up putting it back on within five years.

Another characteristic of these ladies is that they seemed to experience a significant change in their state of mind as they lost their excess weight.

It also became obvious that they all, apparently without exception, were depressed when they considered themselves to be overweight but, as they attempted to lose weight their mood brightened.

For these women, healthy eating became a habit, a habit which then became a normal part of their lives.

They themselves recognized the tremendous role that psychology plays in weight loss.

They refused to look on their efforts to lose weight as a chore but instead chose to have a positive outlook towards their weight loss their new way of eating.

The women also made it a point to chart their progress by weighing themselves regularly.

They also recognized that maintaining weight loss would be a lifetime commitment; they knew that they could not attempt a weight loss program then go back to the old way of eating and exercise.

So if you want to achieve permanent weight loss you must learn new eating patterns that become a way of life for you.

In some ways you could liken your weight loss regime with that of a reformed alcoholic.

You need to recognise that being overweight is not a healthy way to be and, just as the alcoholic must avoid the booze, you must learn to live without whatever it is that causes you to put on weight.

You will probably find that your own weight loss will happen in bursts, at times you may regain some of the lost weight but you must persevere and you will win in the end.

Simply view your setbacks as challenges that you need to overcome.

This may be the key psychological trait that separates successful dieters from unsuccessful ones—perseverance.

In essence, you must change your personality in a positive way in order to achieve your long-term weight loss goals.

Another interesting aspect of this study was that it showed that the women who had undergone weight loss transformation were genuinely happy.

This shows the tremendous psychological impact that weight loss will have on your life.

Once you are free from the burden of extra weight, you will be better able to meet the challenges of life head-on.

And you, the dieter, will benefit from the positive reinforcement you will get as relatives, friends, and co-workers congratulate you for your weight loss.

So, losing weight should be a positive experience and can lead to a more optimistic outlook on life.

It must be noted here that the psychology of weight loss is a complicated matter.

There is no single ingredient that can turn a fat person into a thin one.

However, recognising that there is a psychological component to successful weight loss may, in fact, be half the battle.

Once you recognise that you are engaged in a psychological fight, you are better able to do battle.

By retraining yourself to seek healthy approaches to diet, you can, in effect, transform yourself into a new individual—one that no longer lives to eat, but simply eats to live.

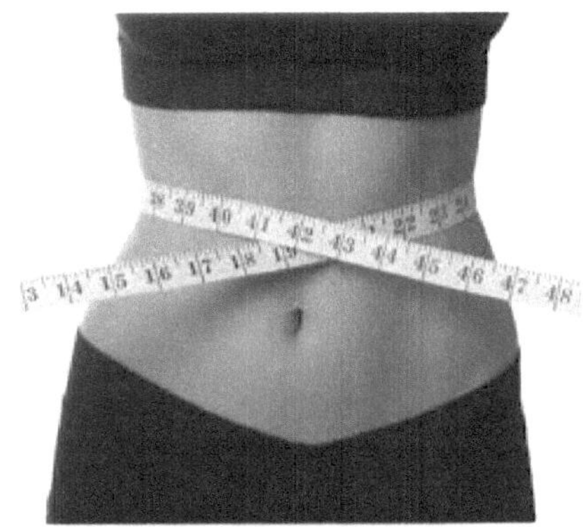

Let's start at the beginning and decide what we mean by "Take Stock"?

We mean, take a good look at yourself, not in terms of your physical appearance, it doesn't matter what you look like at the present time, but you need to assess, as best you can, your abilities, your talents, how you interact with others, your personal preferences and so on.

Once you've "taken stock" you're ready to plan your weight loss diet programme.

With a little research you will be able to list on paper your regular activities, your goals and interests etc. and then work them into a diet and exercise programme that will work for you.

It isn't easy to sit down and do a very honest evaluation of your current condition however it will be very beneficial, not only in terms of your weight loss goals but also with regard to your health in general.

You have to ask yourself some quite hard, searching questions and, this is important, you mustn't "fudge" the answers, after all it's your body and your life which will benefit from the changes which you're about to make.

It's a sobering fact that the second biggest reason behind avoidable deaths, not only in the U.S. but throughout almost the entire developed world, is obesity.

What this means for you of course is that your own evaluation of your own circumstances could possibly have life or death consequences, your life or death!

So take it seriously, be as honest as you can be, enlist the help of those who love you if you're game and write it all down, a week or two down the track you may need to remind yourself why you're doing what you're doing.

Too many weight loss diet plans take a "one size fits all" approach which may work for some people for a while but in the long run are doomed to failure, after all you're unique, your weight loss diet plan needs to fit you and that's why, after you've done your evaluation on yourself you would be well advised to contact a professional dietician and have him or her draw up a weight loss diet plan designed specifically for you.

Take your personal inventory with you when you see your dietician and discuss with him/her your weight loss goals, the areas where you feel you're struggling, where you perhaps need a little more help, how you think you might improve etc..

Tell her/him how long you've been struggling with your weight, whether you seem to be constantly dieting and whether you have the tendency to regain your lost weight after a period of time.

Discuss with your dietician what would be realistic weight loss goals for you, generally if you lose about a kilo each week you're doing well, too much more than that and you're putting an un-necessary strain on yourself, both physically and mentally.

The physical condition of your other family members may also be relevant information which will help your dietician when she/he is working with you to form a good weight loss diet plan.

Just as when you visit your medical practitioner you would tell them of any history in your family of things like heart attacks, diabetes, cancer etc. so you should inform your dietician.

Do you suffer from a high level of cholesterol? Is your blood pressure stable and normal? Are you under any undue stress? Do you get sufficient regular exercise?

These are all legitimate questions which your dietician may ask and you need to be prepared with the answers as far as possible.

Having done all of this with regard to your personal "taking stock" it's important to understand that this has not been done to make you feel bad about yourself but rather to help you and those who will be helping you get a much better idea of where you are now with regard to your health and wellbeing and to plan a course of action to get you to where you want to be.

It's also a good idea to do this exercise every once in a while, say perhaps two or three times a year, so that you can see the progress you're making and perhaps re-evaluate your weight loss goals so that you might achieve even greater success with your diet and exercise program.

As I've said above, taking stock is an important part of your journey to a better, slimmer, fitter you, but having said all of that, "taking stock" is just the beginning, you must now *ACT*, because nothing will change if, at the end of the day you do nothing.

Having taken stock it's time to look at a few reasons why you may be struggling to lose those excess kilos.

You've been a good girl or boy for the last little while, you've been watching what you eat, religiously counting your calories and you've been exercising almost until you drop but you're still not losing too much weight.

You must wonder why?

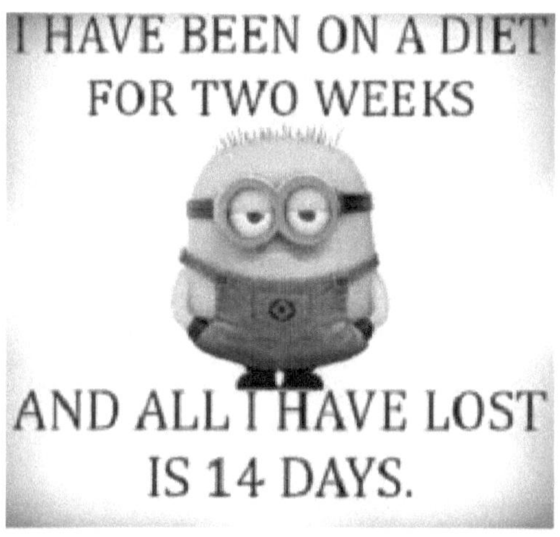

The answer will probably lie with any number of little things you do during your day without even thinking about them, the habits that you wouldn't consider have anything to do with your weight, and much of it begins in your brain.

A marvellous thing the brain, it has the capacity to make things happen with just a thought or two.

For example, when we think of a meal as being "light" our brain will automatically make more ghrelin which is a hormone which increases our appetite.

A study conducted at Yale University concluded that the more ghrelin we produce the less full we feel and this in turn slows our metabolism.

When we're eating "light" we need to focus on the more satisfying elements of the meal, perhaps think more about the cheese and less about the lettuce.

How about the shopping?

Surely how we shop can't have any effect on our weight can it?

Probably not, however it seems that how we pay for our shopping does in fact have some bearing on it.

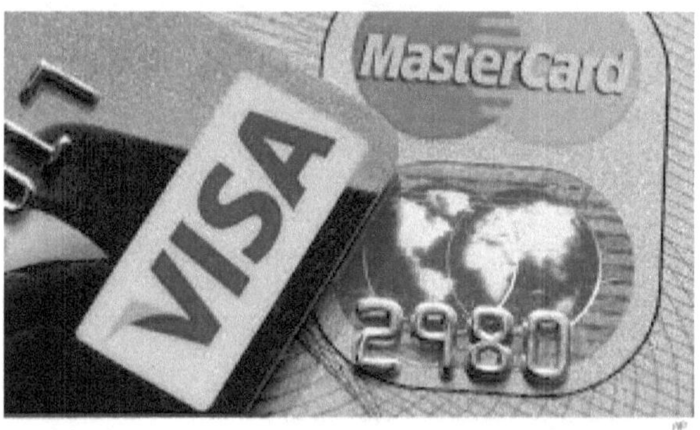

Research has shown that those of us who pay for our groceries with plastic tend to purchase more calorie dense, unhealthy food that those who pay with cash.

According to Dr. Kalpesh Desai, PhD, associate professor of marketing at Binghamton University, it isn't that we're not aware of the choices we make when we shop but it seems that when we don't have to part with cash at the checkout we give in more easily to the impulse of buying junk foods.

Exercising is good, right?

Yes, of course it is, but exercising apparently also has its downside.

A study conducted in France has shown that simply thinking about exercising can cause us to up our food intake by 50%.

Why would this be?

Well, those of us who anticipate our visit to the gym somehow think that the upcoming exercise gives us a licence to snack and we do it without thinking of the consequences.

If we must eat before we hit the treadmill a light snack of less than 150 calories should do us no harm.

Get up and move.

Many of us are prone to sit for periods without getting out of our chairs or away from our workstations and this has a detrimental effect on the way our metabolism works.

When we sit for an extended period of time our bodies stop manufacturing lipase, which is a fat inhibiting enzyme and also our metabolism will slow down.

The American Journal of Clinical Nutrition has found that if we stand up and stretch or go for a short walk at least every hour and we'll increase our metabolism by about 13% and if we fidget all day, say tap our feet or bounce around in our seat we'll burn up to 50% more calories than when we're just sitting.

Get more sleep.

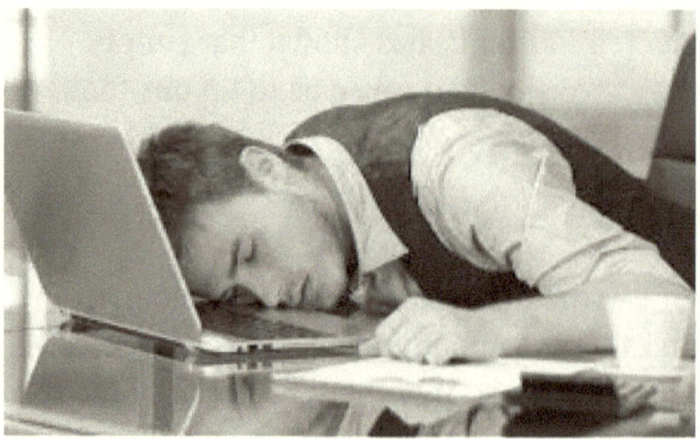

When we don't sleep enough our bodies automatically go into survival mode and there's little we can do about it.

So says Michael Breus, PhD, author of The Sleep Doctor's Diet Plan.

What survival mode does to our bodies is we start to crave fats and carbs and this in turn causes us to put on weight.

A study undertaken by The American Journal of Clinical Nutrition discovered that women who got less than 4 hours sleep consume, on average, 300 more calories and 20 more grams of fat the following day.

Working out how much sleep is enough can sometimes be difficult but a good rule of thumb is when we wake feeling refreshed and ready to go we've had enough sleep, if we wake and feel like we want to turn over and get some more, we haven't.

Feeling stressed?

It seems that stress may have a role to play when it comes to us losing weight.

When we're stressed our bodies produce more cortisol, the stress hormone, and that in turn may increase the amount of fat our bodies store away as visceral fat.

As well as making it difficult to lose weight this visceral fat, which is stored deep in our bodies around the major organs, also increases our risk of developing any number of other very unhealthy conditions including, but not limited to coronary heart disease, cancer, stroke, dementia and so on.

If we can de-stress we will not only make it easier to lose weight but also increase our general wellbeing.

Run or lift weights?

We all know that cardio exercise is important in so many ways but if running, for example, is the only way we get our exercise we aren't doing ourselves any favours when it comes to losing weight.

Who says so?

Jennifer Cohen, the athletic director at the University of Washington and personal trainer to the stars.

Jennifer tells us that if weight loss is our main reason for exercising the we should incorporate some muscle building routines into our exercise program because the more muscle we have the more fat we burn.

If we don't like the weights then some interval training will still be better than cardio alone.

There you have it, just a few reasons why you're perhaps not losing weight.

ARTIFICIAL SWEETENERS.

When we're talking about trying to lose weight one of the subjects that always comes up is that of artificial sweeteners.

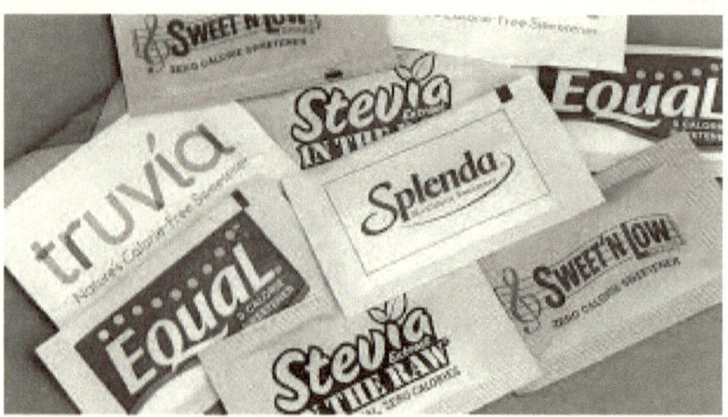

Stevia, aspartame, sucralose, splenda, we've all heard that these, and many other artificial sweeteners, are the bees knees when it comes to weight loss, after all if we cut out the sugar it has to be a good thing doesn't it?

No calories equals instant weight loss right? It has to be good.

BUT, there are some very disturbing facts concerning these products which we need to consider before we embark on the artificial sweetener journey.

First, and this is a good general indication of their worth, artificial sweeteners are one of the foods that nutritionists never eat and there is even some evidence to suggest that they actually cause us to gain weight.

Of 37 studies recently undertaken by scientists at the University of Manitoba into the effects of artificial sweeteners the results indicate that those who use these products had a small but measurable increase in body mass index.

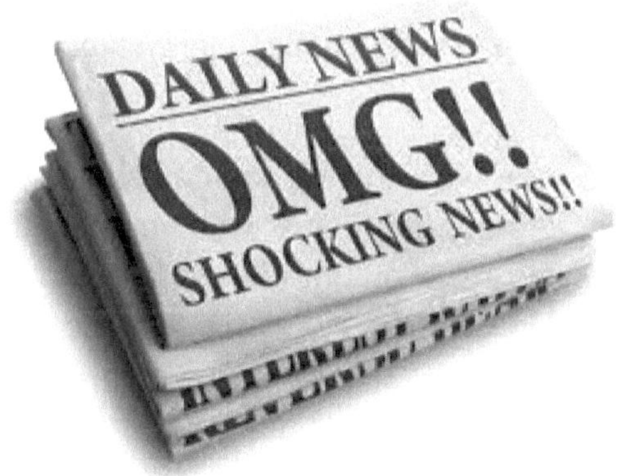

These same studies also show that the use of artificial sweeteners such as stevia, aspartame, sucralose and splenda increase the chances of us developing type 2 diabetes by approximately 14% and should we be long term users we have a 32% increase in the risk of us developing some form of cardiovascular problems.

According to Dr. David Ludwig, an obesity specialist at the Boston Children's Hospital, not all artificial sweeteners are created equal with only five being approved by the FDA in the United States.

These are: Saccharin, acesulfame, aspartame, neotame, and sucralose.

It has also approved one natural low-calorie sweetener, stevia.

There is no scientifically proven reason why artificial sweeteners may be bad for our health but one of the current theories is that when we eat foods which are sweetened artificially we actually increase our body's cravings for the real stuff, we change the way we actually process sugar and we probably change our metabolism for the worse.

Another thought is that we may feel so good about cutting out sugar from our diet that we're tempted to not feel so bad about "cheating" on our diet thus negating the benefits of artificial sweeteners we may otherwise enjoy.

There is also some evidence to suggest that the use of artificial sweeteners may actually change the way we taste our food with many of us who use these products regularly being unable to taste the sweetness in fruit for example and eventually finding unsweetened foods such as vegetables, totally unpalatable.

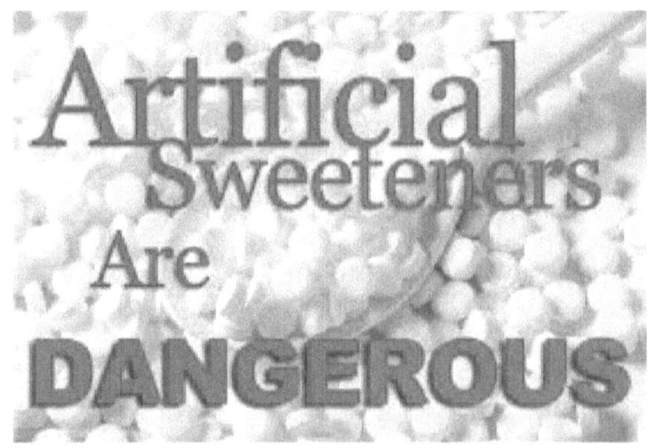

There is also compelling evidence to suggest that artificial sweeteners are highly addictive with animal studies on rats that were previously given cocaine choosing saccharin over cocaine when given the choice.

In people the inclination is to become addicted to overly sweet foods because, as I've said above, unsweetened foods become unpalatable.

Last but by no means least is how we can get those dangerous artificial sweeteners without even knowing it.

We don't have to put saccharin etc. in our coffee to get them, often they are part of the ingredients in a number of other products, there's a partial list below together with a partial list of the most popular artificial sweeteners available today.

Neither of these lists is exhaustive so it is in the interest of our health that we carefully read the label on the products we purchase.

Products That Often Contain Artificial Sweeteners.

Toothpaste and mouthwash

Children's chewable vitamins

Cough syrup and liquid medicines

Chewing gum

No-calorie waters and drinks

Alcoholic beverages

Salad dressings

Frozen yogurt and other frozen deserts

Candies

Baked goods

Yogurt

Breakfast cereals

Processed snack foods

"Lite" or diet fruit juices and beverages

Prepared meats

Nicotine gum

The Most Common Artificial Sweeteners.

Aspartame

Acesulfame potassium

Alitame

Cyclamate

Dulcin

Equal

Glucin

Kaltame

Mogrosides

Neotame

NutraSweet

Nutrinova

Phenlalanine

Saccharin

Splenda

Sorbitol

Sucralose

Twinsweet

Sweet 'N Low

Xylitol

BELLY FAT.

Often when you talk to people about being overweight the issue of "belly fat", fat which accumulates around the tummy area, is the thing that is foremost in their minds.

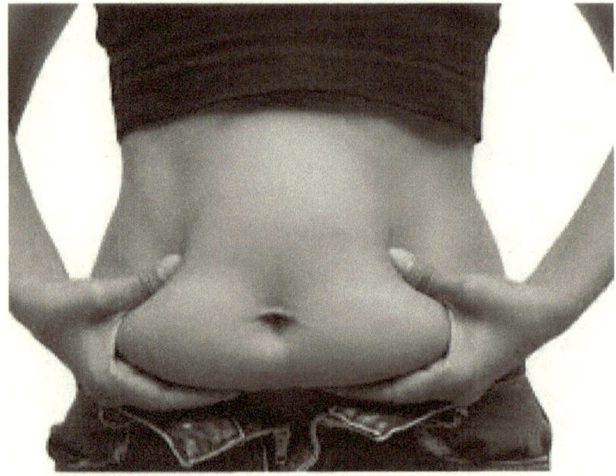

How to lose belly fat is the primary concern of many dieters and it's the main reason many people decide to lose weight in the first place.

If you go to the gym you'll see both men and women working up a sweat by doing abdominal crunches until they exhaust themselves but ab crunches by themselves may make you feel a little better about your efforts but they will do little to get rid of that bothersome belly fat.

In order to reduce belly fat you must first start with what you eat.

You see, you can't effectively lose weight just around your middle, you need to lose it everywhere and the key to doing that is your diet.

It would be nice to be able to choose where the fat comes off from, a little around your butt, some from your thighs etc, but unfortunately it doesn't work like that, your body decides where the weight comes off from not your mind so your job is to slim down everywhere, then you'll see a difference in that "belly fat".

It can get quite disheartening when you see your diet beginning to work but you're losing the weight from perhaps your face first or your arms while that bothersome belly fat stays put.

Apart from deciding to get new parents so that your genes change the only thing you can effectively do is get leaner all over then you can exercise the areas you want to improve, like your abs, to tighten those muscles.

The idea is to improve your diet, eat less processed foods, cut the calories and get your body working again the way it was designed to do.

Then when you hit the gym be selective about what you do.

You see, getting slimmer relies about 90% on your food intake and only 10% on your workouts.

When you do start your exercise programme leave the heavy weights in the rack, go for high repetitions with very little or no weights and do them often.

It's relatively easy to do those ab crunches whenever you have a few spare minutes, you don't have to be dressed in your active wear and lie on an exercise mat, you can sit on a chair and do crunches, I always do mine sitting in bed before I get up in the morning, it's a good way to start your day.

Scientists tell us that "dieting" alone won't get rid of that belly fat permanently; you may be able to lose some of that weight initially but almost 3/4 of dieters regain their lost weight, and then some, within 3-5 years.

This is because most people, when they think of "dieting" they imagine some of the extremes which are bandied about.

Living on half a lettuce leaf and 2 small carrots a day may, no will, make you lose weight but it isn't all that healthy is it?

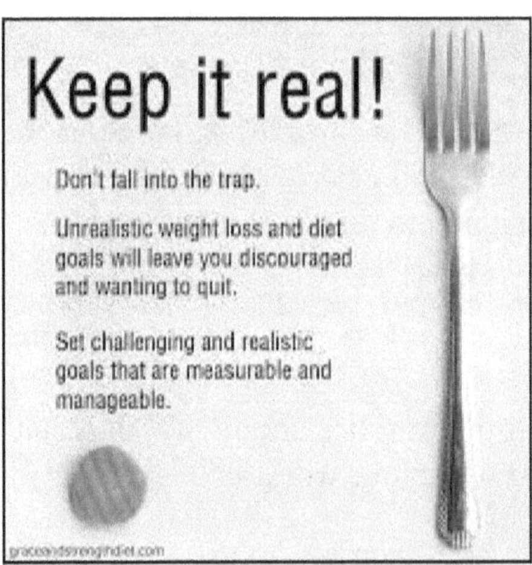

Likewise the eating fads you are likely to read about in some of the less reputable women's magazines; those which may be promoted as fast weight loss programmes are great for the celebrity who needs to lose some kilos for their latest film role but are not the way for you and I to lose weight permanently without damaging our health.

A long term solution is one that will help you to reduce the number of calories you take in without leaving you feeling like you're going to faint from a lack of food or be left with no energy to go about your normal daily routine.

The proven best solution is to stop eating before you start to feel full.

The people who live on the Japanese island of Okinawa live the longest of any people on the planet and they have a philosophy which they call "hara hachi bun me", roughly translated it says "eat only until you are 80 % full."

That's a good way to be when you're losing weight.

Eating until you're not quite full takes a little self control, especially if you've been an over-eater in the past but it is something which you can do with a little effort, it is important, however, not to snack between your meals because you don't feel satisfied, that defeats the whole purpose.

Just to summarise, when it comes to losing that belly fat you can't just exercise it away.

The primary temptation of most of us is to try to work it off, we tend to hit the gym, pump the iron, crunch the abs, run until our legs are like jelly, after all, who has ever seen a long distance runner with belly fat?

The reality of it is that a flat stomach has more to do with low body fat all over and that only comes from a combination of the correct eating plan plus exercise.

As exasperating as it is the only way you're going to turn your belly fat into something to be proud of is to find the right diet, one that works for you, be consistent with it and do your exercises regularly.

Patience is the key, the results won't happen overnight but if you do it right the results will be sustainable in the long term and you will have defeated the dreaded "belly fat" forever.

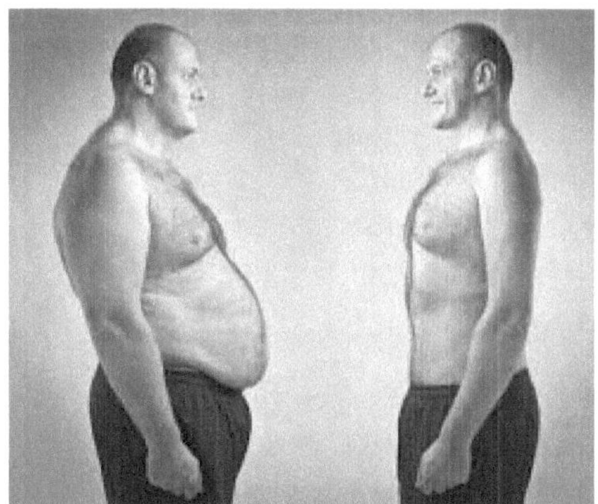

As we get older it should be no surprise that our bodies don't have the same capacity to "bounce back" as they did in our youth.

When we look in the mirror in the morning and see bags under our eyes and wrinkles where there once was smooth beautiful skin we start to see this.

Then we get dressed and find that those pants that fitted so comfortably are now a little tight around the middle and suddenly we realise that the dreaded "belly fat" has arrived in our lives.

Belly fat, the bane of many people's lives and the subject of much discussion especially in the health magazines and web blogs.

When I ask people what is the most pressing concern they have concerning their weight the answer [almost always] is the fat that has accumulated around their middle, the dreaded "belly fat".

Not only does the appearance of belly fat mean our clothes don't fit as comfortably as they once did or we don't look as slim and svelte as we used to, belly fat also brings with it some health concerns which we don't need.

According to the Mayo Clinic, belly fat is not just limited to the extra fat just below the skin, it also gives rise to unhealthy fat which sits deep inside your body and surrounds your internal organs.

Having a large amount of belly fat increases your risk of a number of very unhealthy conditions such as heart disease, type 2 diabetes, high blood pressure, cancer of the colon, sleep apnoea and premature death from any number of other causes.

I guess it would be fair to say that I don't need it and neither do you!

So the question is "how do I get rid of the belly fat?"

While the question is easy I'm afraid the answer isn't so easy.

The bad news is that belly fat, the fat which accumulates around our middle can't be reduced or eliminated on its own.

It has been proven that the "spot reduction" of fat from our bodies just isn't possible, we can't slim down our bellies or our thighs or our upper arms without reducing the excess fat from the rest of our body as well.

When we start to lose weight it's our genetics that decide where that weight will disappear from first.

For most of us the weight comes of in a reasonably even fashion, a little from here, a little from there, but some of us have a nasty tendency to store what's called "visceral" fat, that's fat which is stored deep inside our bodies and surrounds our internal organs.

This "visceral fat" means that for those of us who store it, as I said above, it's a health disaster just waiting to happen.

Continuing with the "bad news", we can't do 200 ab crunches a day and expect to eliminate the belly fat, it just doesn't happen that way, we need to lose weight from all over, increase our metabolism by getting more exercise and eating healthier foods and don't expect immediate results.

By all means do the crunches, they won't do us any harm but persist with the lifestyle changes and given a little time we will see that dreaded belly fat just slowly melt away, not only will we look great when it's gone but we'll feel much better for it.

CARBS.

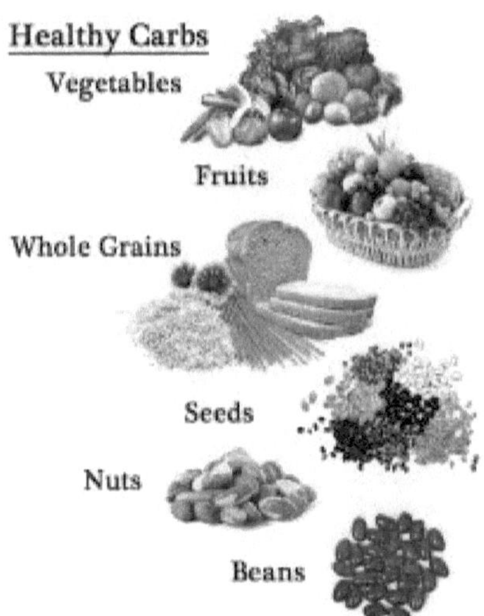

Carbs, or carbohydrates as they are more correctly known, are well known to everyone who has tried to lose weight.

There are a number of low carb diet plans floating around which are based on the assumption that carbs are what cause a great deal of excess weight and that they should be eliminated from our diet altogether or at least eaten in very limited amounts.

Nothing could be further from the truth.

We see, not all carbohydrates are created equal.

With most things in life there is good and bad and carbohydrates are no different, there are good carbohydrates and there are bad carbohydrates and while it is true that we can lose weight by cutting down on the carbs, carbs are an essential part of a healthy diet.

We get carbs from almost any food which we consume, bread and pasta, fruit and vegetables all contain carbs and carbs come indifferent forms, they come in the form of sugars, starches and even fibre so we see, to avoid carbs altogether is no easy task and is completely un-necessary, even unhealthy.

The human digestive system has been carefully designed to deal with carbs, it generally transforms them into blood sugar or glucose which then provides the energy our bodies need to perform the functions which allow us to live our lives as we would like.

Fatigue can often be traced back to a lack of sufficient carbohydrates in our bodies because carbs are full of other nutrients, vegetables are a good source of vitamins and fibre, fruit is full of vitamins A and C as well as folate, whole grains, not so much the processed variety, contain protein, vitamin B and, of course, fibre and legumes give us protein, potassium and iron.

So we see carbs are essentially good for our health, *but* that doesn't apply to *all carbs.*

Potato chips, biscuits [cookies] and soft drinks like Coke, lemonade etc. also contain carbs in the form of flour and sugar and these aren't good for us at all.

These carbs are very high in calories, contain little by way of nutrients, have next to no fibre so cannot keep we satisfied and will have us coming back for more in no time.

Refined carbohydrates have also been linked to diabetes and heart disease which makes them a dangerous choice and gives us a good reason to ban them from our diet, quite apart from the fact that most of them will only help us to gain weight not lose it.

The truth is that these types of carbs will give us nothing by way of nutrients but plenty in the form of fat, not really what we want.

If we avoid most processed grains and sugars and instead choose to eat whole grains, vegetables and fruit we will be making the most of our intake of nutrients without jeopardising our waistline.

There are some reliable estimates that suggest that about 75% of overweight people are actually addicted to carbohydrates.

This is a dangerous situation because it can suggest that these people have too much insulin in their system and that in turn prompts them to eat the wrong types of food and to eat it often.

Some of the indications of carb addiction are mood swings, un-reasonable fatigue and even migraines caused by low blood sugar.

Eating a whole bag of potato chips in one sitting or half of that beautiful cake we just made could also be an indication of a carb addiction.

When we become addicted to carbs we actually have conditioned our body to consume as many carbs as it can and therefore it seems that no matter how much we eat we're never really satisfied.

There is something called "The Official Carb Addicts Plan", [I really don't know how "official" it is] that suggests that we eat a meal made up of protein and vegetables [meat or fish and two or three veg] twice a day and protein and carb and starch free vegetables for the third meal.

This plan even allows for a small dessert after our third meal which they call a reward meal.

The authors of this plan think that if we skip the carbs for two of our three meals a day we will eventually lose the craving for those unhealthy carbs.

If you think that you may be addicted to carbs you can get more information on the "Official Carb Addicts Plan" by following the link.

CHILDHOOD OBESITY.

Have you ever watched a group of children playing together and wondered why half of them seem to be overweight and perhaps as many as half of that half could probably be considered obese?

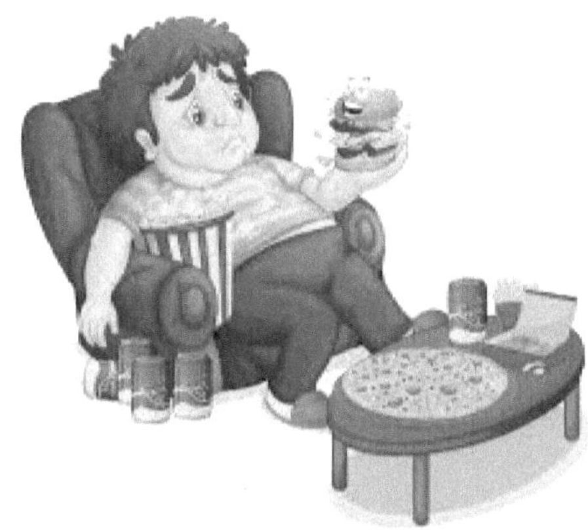

Childhood obesity is a reasonably recent health dilemma and it's one which is difficult to manage especially when every parent wants to make sure that their children are well nourished and healthy.

It's obvious that many obese children shed the excess weight as they grow into adulthood but it's equally as obvious that many do not and whether it's an adult or a child that is over-weight each can, and probably will, suffer feelings of general displeasure with life, perhaps feeling unworthy of the good things life has to offer and almost certainly feeling unshakable tiredness throughout the day.

Childhood obesity also increases the risk of heart disease and diabetes later in life.

The relative authority in the USA has deduced that over the last thirty or so years the number of children with major weight related issues has doubled with no regard to age, background or ethnic group, it's affecting ALL young people.

It seems that obese children are less inclined to be socially engaged than their peers, they will often have difficulty making and keeping friends, they are at risk of becoming loners making them the prime candidates for our "lost generation".

Most will feel that their weight is out of control but they don't know what to do about it and their parents will often not realise just how serious the problem of childhood obesity is, indeed many will take great offense if they are told, even by their medical professional, that their child is obese.

It's not unusual for parents of obese children to be obese themselves nor is it unusual for them to consider obesity in their children to be just a passing thing which will go away as they grow.

They will often fail to see the evidence of their own struggles with weight or to equate it to the condition of their offspring.

So what causes childhood obesity?

The answer to that question is for more qualified people than me to answer however there does seem to be a small number of readily recognisable triggers which point to possible causes.

With the pace of life being so fast these days it's an unfortunate fact that many families aren't able to find the time to sit down as a family and eat a balanced meal,

McDonalds, KFC, Hungry Jacks and the like have become the stand in dinner providers and as a consequence the younger generation are getting too much fat and sugar and not enough real goodness in their food.

When asked, many parents believe that their children's diets are less healthy than were theirs when they were young.

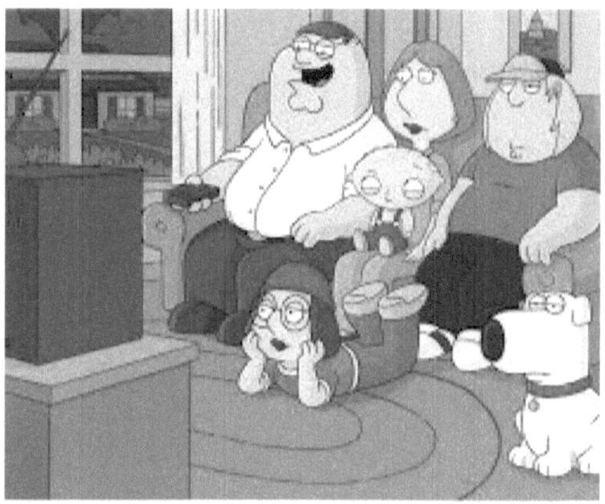

Computers and television are other major contributing factors with many children spending more than 25 hours each week in front of the TV and almost as many hours in front of a computer screen.

This means, of course, that the outside, run around playtime which the older generation enjoyed during their younger years is missing to a great extent for our children and with it the fat burning exercise which was inherent in that pursuit.

Perhaps it's also important to recognise that when we are overweight, as adults or as children, we find it difficult to take part in even the most leisurely of sporting activities.

Without some good encouragement it's easier to sit on the sidelines and watch others run and jump than it is to actually get involved.

Advertising can also have a detrimental effect on the weight of young people.

Children are especially influenced by adverts, many of which are aimed squarely in their direction.

Craving the things which they see advertised on television and elsewhere, children will not recognise the dangers in foods loaded with sugar and fat, it then becomes the responsibility of their parents to monitor what they eat and often parents are too busy or are unaware of the nutritional content, or lack of it, of the food in their refrigerators.

Childhood obesity is a modern day problem and it is a serious one, but fortunately it is a problem which can be quite easily overcome.

Encourage your younger family members to take up a sport or perhaps learn to dance, go with them to their training, dance with them in your lounge room with the music turned up a bit, if you live close take them to the beach for a swim or just a brisk walk in the soft sand.

It isn't difficult to get some exercise for yourself as well as for your child if you put your mind to it.

TV time for children and teenagers is, for the most part, wasted time with nothing to recommend it so give some thought to limiting the amount of time they spend watching TV or playing their computer games but don't stop it altogether or you will just make them resentful, if you find them something else to do which is just as interesting [that shouldn't be too difficult] you'll find that they will gradually wean themselves off.

Likewise with food, with a little encouragement from you and some experimentation at dinner time your young ones will soon come to prefer the good, wholesome, tasty food which you serve up instead of the fast junk food which they may be used to.

This all takes some work on your part but to see your child grow into a healthy adult with no weight problems and no health problems caused by being overweight as a child will make the effort well worth it.

DON'T EAT OUT!

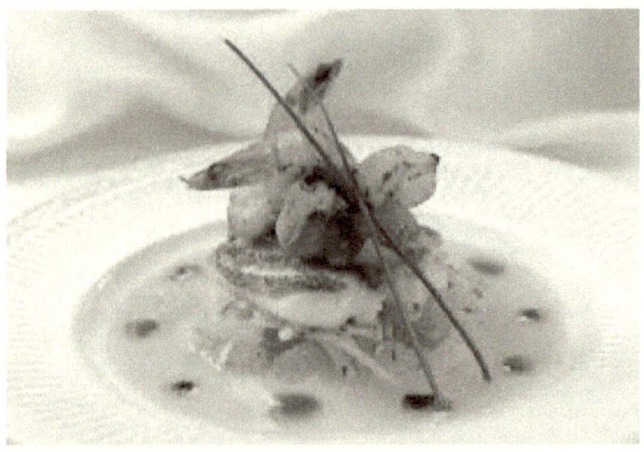

When we're looking to lose weight recent research suggests that a home cooked meal is better for our waistline than a meal eaten in a restaurant.

Many of us like to eat out, myself included, but spending an evening or two eating at a restaurant is doing us no favours when it comes to our weight says Dr. Caroline Cederquist, a weight management specialist.

Dr. Cederquist discovered that in the late 1970s about 80% of our calories were consumed at home but by 2015 that figure had dropped to approximately 40% and the obesity rate [in the USA] during that same period had climbed dramatically with more than 70 percent of the adult population now overweight or obese.

These same figures are approximately appropriate for children and it's an alarming statistic.

Why does restaurant prepared food have so many more calories than the food we prepare at home?

We need to remember that restaurants are in the business of making money not helping us to lose weight, in order to do that they must make their food as tasty and enjoyable as they can and this means relying much more on salt, sugar and cooking oils and fats.

Restaurants also tend to deliver a larger portion size than we might possibly serve at home and many serve bread before or with the meal making healthy food choices more difficult.

What about those entrées we all love to get stuck into while we're waiting for our main meal to appear, well they can be a diet killer all on their own.

A side dish of fried onion rings can contain a whopping 2000 calories while a bread starter alone can contain upwards of 500 calories and that's without the dip and while we're unlikely to eat all of the appetiser on our own we are still going consume a decent portion of it and get the calories as well.

Now very few of us will eat out without also having something to drink and while water with the meal is a good idea the soda or beer isn't.

A standard drink of soda, or soft drink as we call it in Oz, contains about 150 calories, a regular beer is about the same whereas a glass of wine is only slightly less at about 130 calories.

All of a sudden the calorie count in our restaurant meal is climbing out of control and we haven't considered the main course yet.

If you're anything like me you'll love those sauces the restaurant chefs love to put on just about everything but they all push the calorie count into the stratosphere.

Well I guess we can always order a salad can't we?

Consider this, a salad with 2 cups of lettuce or spinach, 1/2 cup of sliced carrots, a cup of cherry tomatoes and 2 tablespoons of fat-free Italian dressing has about 100 calories [but who would want to eat it?].

Add a 1/2 cup of grilled chicken and you're adding just 61 calories, but if you choose fried chicken instead, you'll add 194 calories.

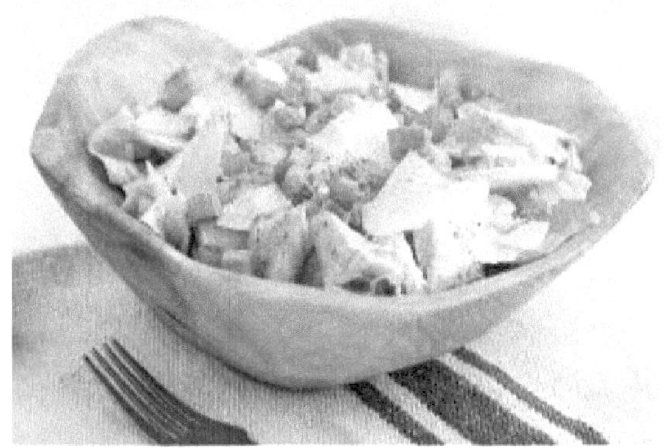

Not too bad, however if we decide to replace it with traditional Caesar salad we get almost 500 calories, 40 grams of fat (9 grams of which are saturated) and 1070 milligrams of sodium.

Perhaps Caesar salad isn't our answer!

What about the smorgasbord or buffet, we get to choose what we put on our plate and how much and how often we go back for more, what a good idea.

But it's only a good idea if we can limit ourselves to eating those items which are part of our diet plan and only eating the correct portions, if we are able to do that then we're onto a good thing but resisting the temptation is not so easy for many of us, that's how we got to be overweight in the first place.

By now our diet is blown and we haven't got to dessert yet.

Eating out of course doesn't only mean eating in a restaurant, how often do we buy something to eat while we're driving or sitting in the car with a loved one watching the sun set?

That can also be a trap, much of the food we purchase as take away or food to go is deep fried, the British favourite of fish and chips is a prime example.

I love it but it has so many calories that I can't count that high and most take away food is the same, loaded with fat and designed to kill our diet stone dead.

So what's the answer if we're unable to avoid eating away from home?

Stick to the plan, don't indulge, not even just once because we know it won't be just once, select food which we know won't cause us a problem, limit the size of the portion we eat even if we need to bag the remainder and take it with us for our next meal and stay in control.

Our stomachs will thank us for it, our waistlines will thank us for it and we'll still be on the right track when we wake up in the morning.

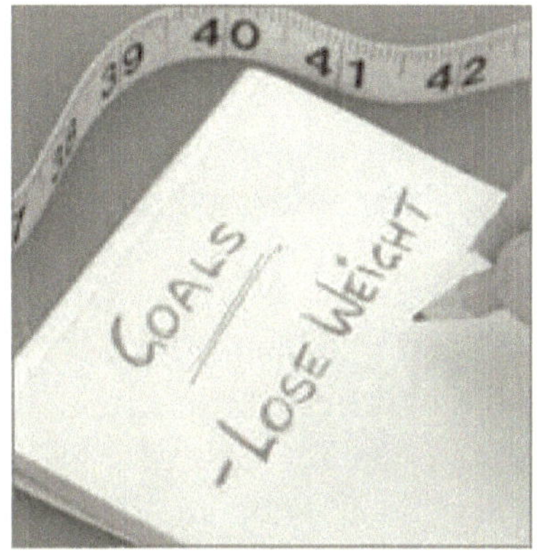

We all know that losing weight isn't easy, some of us have been on the weight loss treadmill for years, losing weight today only to put it back on tomorrow.

Every time we go out to do the grocery shopping we're confronted with the wonderful smell of bread baking in the local bakery, we stop to have coffee and there are all those delicious pastries just put there on display to tempt us.

If we've been overweight for some time then it's very hard to put aside the habits of a lifetime and do things differently into the future.

Here are some of the most difficult dietary habits we need to overcome if we are to reach our weight loss goals.

Weight Loss Sabotage 1 - Snacking Between Meals.

Now getting peckish between meals isn't unusual, nor is it completely avoidable, but what we eat when we do get hungry between meals is within our control and how we snack is very important when it comes to achieving our weight loss goals.

Munchies that contain high amounts of fibre are good for us that like to snack between meals.

I am, by nature, a "grazer", I like to eat throughout the day not just at meal times and I find that if I eat the much of the snack food that I find on the supermarket shelf or in most coffee shops it does my waist line no good at all.

Snacks like popcorn, potato chips, sweet biscuits [cookies] all contain either high amounts of sugar or salt and plenty of calories, in fact very little which will help our diet.

High fibre snacks will help us to feel fuller for longer and thereby reduce the feeling that we need to eat more.

<u>Weight Loss Sabotage 2 - Dining Out.</u>

Dining out at a good restaurant is one of life's more enjoyable pleasures but when we do eat at a good restaurant it does us well to remember that the restaurant is in the business of selling food that tastes good not helping us to lose weight.

Often that means that the food we get served will have a little too much salt or sugar or fat of some kind.

These things all tend to increase the flavour of the food making it taste good but they do us more harm than good when it comes to controlling our weight.

By all means go to your favourite restaurant just don't go there too often.

<u>Weight Loss Sabotage 3 - Boredom.</u>

I don't know about you but when I'm bored I tend to head to the fridge.

Now boredom, as you well know, is caused by having nothing to do, nothing of any worth to think about and in that state our brain releases a neurotransmitter called dopamine which is in charge of our feelings of pleasure amongst other things.

According to http://www.news-medical.net -

"Dopamine is the chemical that mediates pleasure in the brain. It is released during pleasurable situations and stimulates one to seek out the pleasurable activity or occupation. This means food, sex, and several drugs of abuse are also stimulants of dopamine release in the brain, particularly in areas such as the nucleus accumbens and prefrontal cortex."

That may mean as little to you as it does to me however it does to some degree explain why I, and possibly you, seek out food when we're bored, it stimulates the release of dopamine and as a result makes us feel good.

Does that mean that we shouldn't eat when we're bored?

Probably not, but we should be careful about what we eat, leave the potato chips, the biscuits, the lollies alone and go for something which is healthy and non fattening instead.

Perhaps this is a good time to ask ourselves if we're really hungry, if we're not then chewing some gum or drinking a glass of water would be a better option.

<u>Weight Loss Sabotage 4 - Skipping Meals.</u>

Skipping meals may seem to make sense when we're trying to lose weight, after all the less food we consume the fewer calories we have to deal with during our periods of exercise.

This, however, is not the case.

Missing meals, especially breakfast, means:

• we don't kick start our metabolism at the beginning of the day

• we deprive our bodies of the essential nutrients they need to function effectively

• we suffer from poor concentration and fatigue throughout the day

• we will tend to overeat at other meal times.

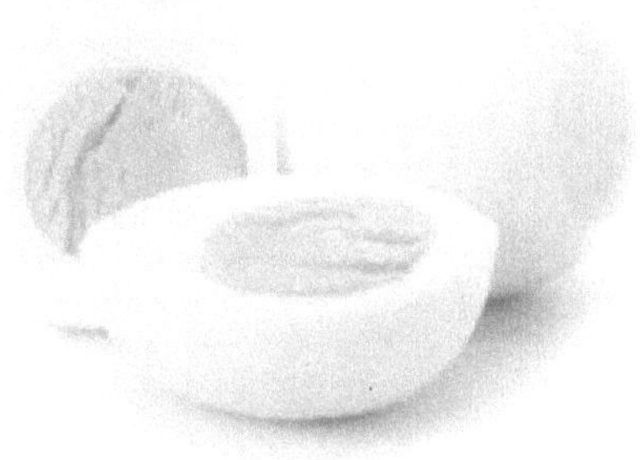

A good breakfast is one of the best ways to start our day and eggs, including the yolk, are perhaps the very best food to have at the beginning of our day.

Demonized by many in the past for their high cholesterol, eggs are chock full of essential nutrients like vitamins A and B12, selenium and phosphorus.

One large egg has only about 80 calories, contains perhaps six grams of protein and will put us on the right track for a great day without putting on any weight just don't combine it with other less healthy foods like bacon fried in lots of fat or a bagel and cheese.

[A bagel typically has about 250 calories, has 15% sodium and 20% protein].

These are just a few ways in which we can very effectively kill any chance we might have of losing weight.

As I said above losing weight isn't easy, everyone who's ever been overweight knows that, stay away from these bad dietary habits and don't sabotage your own weight loss goals.

64

EMOTIONAL EATING.

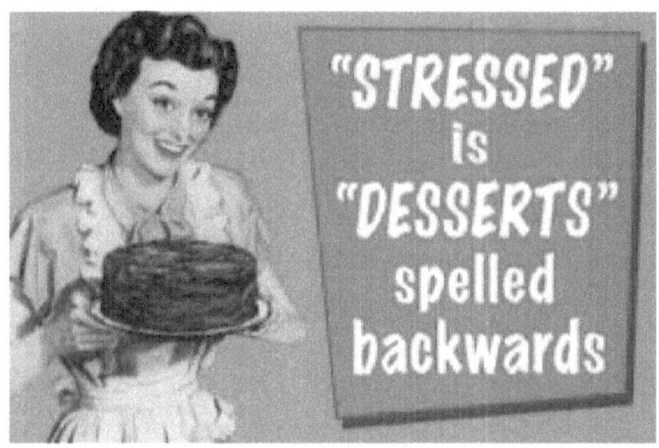

Are you an emotional eater?

Before answering that question we need to know what an "emotional eater" is.

Emotional eating, according to those who are supposed to know these things, is eating as a result of something which is happening in your life which is related in some way to your mental or emotional state rather than eating because you are, or think you should be, hungry.

Modern thinking regarding unwanted weight gain puts most of the blame firmly on eating as a way to relieve some of the stresses of life.

This applies to both men and women and so called "comfort food" is to blame.

Anxiety, depression, significant loss, even plain old boredom can cause us to raid the fridge or the cookie jar to get a fix of this comfort food.

When you can't be bothered to go and exercise or do that job in the yard that's been waiting for days, or weeks, sometimes it's just easier to make a coffee, grab a doughnut and chill.

When you're depressed you may think that you have nothing better to do than eat and that eating, emotional eating, can easily lead to weight gain which in turn can cause more depression, it becomes a vicious circle which can be hard to break.

So, are you an emotional eater?

How do you tell?

You need to ask yourself some key questions and give yourself the honest answers.

Do you have a tendency to eat when you're sad?

When things get you down, when you're overly concerned about something, when you're scared?

Do you use food, especially very sweet or fatty food, when you need a lift or after you've had a disappointment?

Does food help you to deal with some of the more unpleasant things which you have to face from time to time?

If you've answered "yes" to any of these questions, or others like them, you may well be eating to help you deal with the emotional issues associated with them.

If you have indeed identified yourself as an emotional eater the next step is to accept that fact, much as an alcoholic needs to accept that he or she is an alcoholic, you can then begin to deal with it.

The most effective way to do this is to use a diversionary tactic.

When you're down and you consider going to the kitchen for a comforting snack find something else to do instead.

Go for a walk around the yard or down the street, pick up the needles and start to knit that new jumper for yourself, or crochet a new blanket, that would take your mind off food for a while.

You'll find that as you start to become involved with something else the thought of food will just fade into the background or even disappear altogether.

Another thing you should do is to identify the things that start the food cravings or the regular times when you tend to "over-snack".

Do you eat while you're watching TV in the evenings, while you're mentally engaged in something, while you're reading etc.?

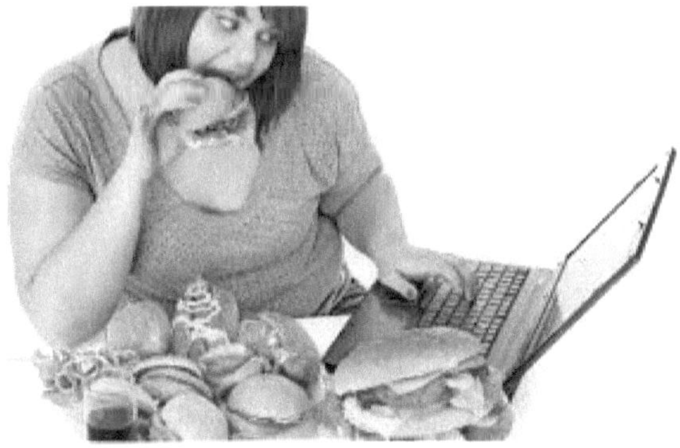

When you know the answers to these questions you can more easily work out a strategy to change your behaviour patterns to those which don't involve eating or snacking.

Also, just as with any other emotional issue, it will help if you have a support network of those who care about your health and wellbeing.

This network could be made up of your immediate family, your work colleagues, your social group or perhaps even others who are in the same situation as yourself.

You might even consider joining a support group who specialise in helping those who want to slim down.

Whenever you feel the need to get stuck into the snacks you could contact someone in your support team for a little, well, support!

Should you find that you are eating because you are depressed or particularly anxious it is important to seek out professional help.

Your medical professional is the place to go for help to overcome those feelings, depression is something that shouldn't be taken lightly or treated as inconsequential, professional help is never far away and seeking it is the proper course of action under those circumstances.

If your depression becomes severe there will be organisations run by both your government and private sources which are specifically there to help those in that situation, seek their help, don't try to deal with it on your own, in Australia it's called "Beyond Blue" their phone number is 1300 22 4636

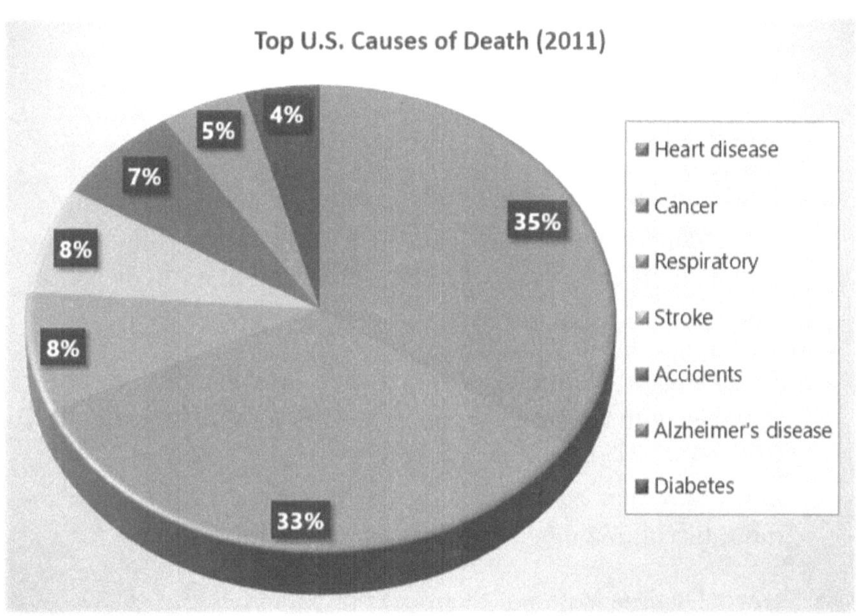

We all know that if we're carrying more weight than we should it affects our health.

Overweight people can't do many of the things that others take for granted, things like going for a long walk or playing football with the kids in the park but how many of us understand that being overweight can increase our risk of developing up to 50 different health problems.

That's not a typo, obese people and even those who are overweight but not technically obese have a greater risk of a huge number of unwanted health problems including heart disease, gallstones, stroke, certain cancers, diabetes and even depression.

A study undertaken at Harvard University over a period of 10 years combined the results from 120,000 women and 50,000 men and revealed some very alarming statistics about the relationship between weight and health.

Those who volunteered to take part in the study provided the researchers with details of their weight and height as well as their eating and exercise habits and their medical history.

Their general wellbeing was recorded over that period together with the fluctuations in their BMI and the results showed a direct relationship between their body mass index and their general health, the higher the BMI the more likelihood there was for them to suffer disease.

Heart Disease is one of the most prevalent health problems of the modern age, much of it is caused by us carrying excess weight and much of it is preventable.

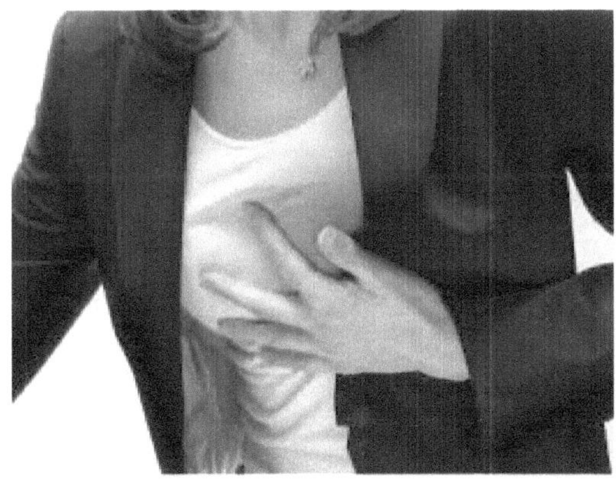

Together with stroke, heart disease and other cardiovascular issues are responsible, according to the American Heart Association, for over 800,000 deaths per year in the United States alone, that's one life lost every 40 seconds, over 2200 every day, that is a very sobering statistic.

That's just in the US, worldwide the figure must be enormous!

How is this related to our excess weight or obesity?

When we are overweight our blood pressure rises and we tend to accumulate unhealthy levels of bad fats and cholesterol in our blood, both being precursors to heart disease and stroke.

Overweight people are about six times more likely to have high blood pressure than those of us who are a little leaner, again, according to the American Heart Association, when we carry an extra 10 kilos [that's about 22 lbs] of weight the increase caused to our blood pressure increases our risk of stroke by a huge 24%.

Makes you think....

What About Diabetes?

Diabetes is so closely linked to excess weight that many clinicians have now coined the phrase "diabesity" to describe the condition.

Almost 90% of people with type 2 diabetes, [that includes me], are overweight or obese.

In the last 30 years the incidence of type 2 diabetes has risen by about 65% and many believe this is caused by a poor diet with too much sugar and bad fats such as is found in fast foods.

The high blood sugar level which is characteristic of type 2 diabetes is also a cause of metabolic syndrome, a group of conditions which, when occurring together increase our risk of heart disease, stroke and diabetes.

Metabolic syndrome also carries with it, if left untreated, a number of other very worrying health problems such as blindness, kidney failure and foot or leg amputations.

Diabetes related health conditions are currently the seventh leading cause of death in the United States.

And Cancer.....

Many of us don't associate obesity with cancer but it's uncomfortable to learn that obesity is the second leading cause of cancer in the developed world, beaten only by cigarette smoking.

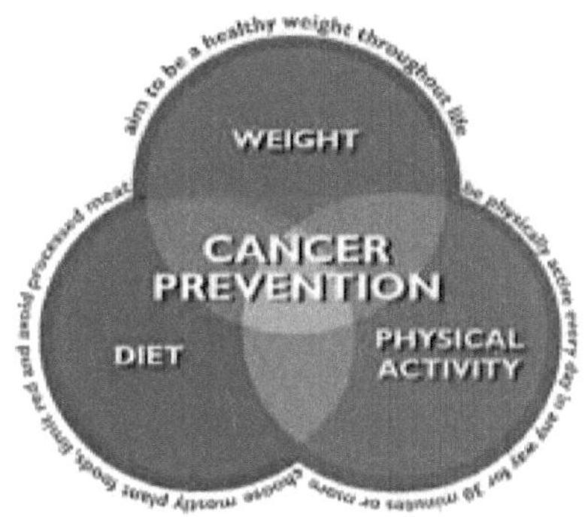

The American Cancer Society conducted a 15 year long study of almost 1 million people and concluded that carrying excess weight is a factor in the formation of many different types of cancer.

Those over 50 years of age are in the firing line, particularly if they are overweight, with something in the order of 14% of men and up to 20% of women who die from a cancer related illness having it attributed to obesity.

Both men and women who have a higher than healthy BMI have a correspondingly higher risk of dying from cancers of the kidney, gallbladder, liver, rectum and colon, pancreas and oesophagus while in women the risk of uterus, ovarian, cervical and breast cancer also increased and in men, cancers of the stomach or prostate were also indicated.

Perhaps part of the problem with obesity and cancer is that those of us who are obese tend to shy away from visiting our doctor for the necessary screening and other tests, possibly because of some degree of discomfort at being subjected to physically invasive and at times uncomfortable examinations.

Depression is also a major effect of being overweight.

Here we have a "chicken and egg" question, are we depressed because we are overweight or are we overweight because we're depressed?

A number of scientific studies have found that either scenario is likely to be true with over 50% of obese people at a higher risk of becoming depressed over time when compared to people of healthy weight.

Obesity can have the effect of changing our brain chemistry because of the stress it causes us but peer pressure and the "thin is beautiful" culture which surrounds us today may also play a part.

When we see ourselves being fatter than those beautiful people who we come into contact with every day our self-esteem is affected in a negative way and this is known to be a major cause of depression.

Eating disorders and the physical discomfort which comes with being overweight are also triggers for depression and according to a 2010 study in the Archives of General Psychiatry almost 60% of people with depression risk becoming obese.

When we're depressed we're also less inclined to eat properly and exercise is often just too much bother which just adds to the weight gain cycle.

Lastly we need to remember that some medications which are prescribed to treat depression will actually cause us to put on weight so it's a good idea to discuss this with your doctor when she/he is about to prescribe your antidepressants.

NB Please be aware that I am not a medical professional and this article is given for your information only, if you have problems with depression or any other medical condition please see your doctor and stay healthy.

DON'T FORGET TO EXERCISE.

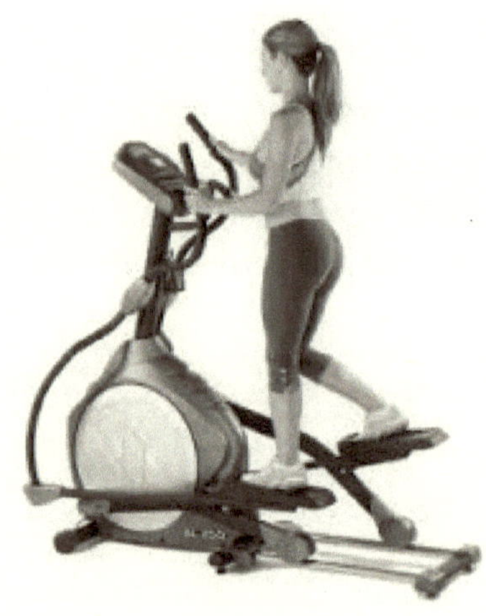

If you believe all that you read on the 'net, 50% of people who want to lose weight don't actually do any, or very little, exercise.

That is a startling assertion considering that regular exercise is a core part of any serious weight loss programme however it really isn't that surprising when you think about it.

Exercise was part of everyday life for almost everyone in times gone by.

Before the invention of all the labour saving devices we have access to now everything was done "the hard way".

The farmer had to work his land without a tractor, the housewife did the washing by hand, students had to walk to school and so on.

Everyday life for the majority of people involved some form of regular exercise.

Before the worker went out for the day he or she had a good breakfast to sustain them and when they got home at night a hearty meal was waiting, and needed, to replenish their energy.

There was no need for a regular exercise programme apart from that.

Today things are different, most workers sit to do their daily chores, the farmer sits on his tractor, the housewife loads the washing machine and the kids get a ride to school.

Don't misunderstand me, I know that many people still work hard, I know that being a housewife, for example, isn't an easy job but it really doesn't involve the physical activity which our mothers and grandmothers had to undertake.

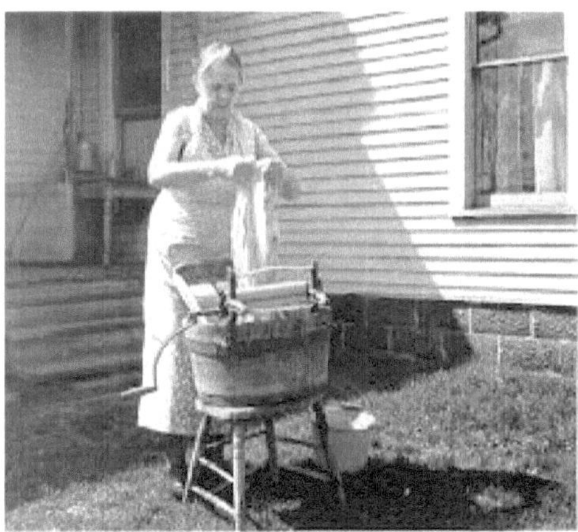

Even the lack of exercise in our daily lives wouldn't be so much of a problem if we had changed our eating habits to match the change in our daily exercise routine but we haven't.

When we've been at work all day we still expect to come home to something reasonably substantial to eat don't we?

After all we've worked hard all day and we're hungry but the work we've done for the most part isn't physical labour and it hasn't resulted in us expending lots of energy which now needs replacing.

Most of us don't get the opportunities to exercise that our forebears got and so we must take the initiative and find ways to exercise, to move and stretch our limbs, to flex our muscles the way they were designed to.

Sitting in front of the television or computer just doesn't do it.

While it is important to reduce your calorie intake if you want to lose weight the very best weight loss programmes combine a sensible diet with regular exercise.

Exercise has proven to be the best way to boost your metabolism and that is one of the key ingredients to your weight loss success.

In order to lose the kilos you need to burn an incredible amount of calories so combining exercise with reducing your calorie intake offers you the very best chance of weight loss success.

So what do you do if you don't enjoy exercising, how can you get motivated to even begin let alone stay with it?

Well one good way is to find someone to exercise with.

A reliable friend who will regularly join you in your exercise programme is a good start, perhaps getting your children involved by playing some backyard sport with them once or twice a week, if you're a new mum then take your newborn for a jog in the stroller, you could even join a local walking or exercise group if that's you.

If "exercise" doesn't float your boat then look for something you really enjoy and base your exercise around that.

Perhaps you enjoy a social game of tennis or golf [leave the buggy in the shed and walk the course], if rock and roll is your thing then pump up the volume while you do your housework, you'll find yourself jigging around the house.

What you do is not nearly as important as that you do it and do it regularly.

Even, dare I say it, sex is good exercise, spice up your sex life and make your partner happy to be a part of your exercises ;-).

If you can afford it a personal trainer is a good idea, research shows us that those who engage a personal trainer will have more weight loss success than those who choose to go it alone.

Whichever route you decide to take make daily exercise a part of your regular routine, it should come as naturally as sitting down to dinner each evening because the truth is you need regular exercise to maintain a healthy mind as well as a healthy body.

To help us all to get as much exercise as we can I've investigated a number of "exercise machines" which we can use at home whenever we have a spare minute or two and on the following pages you'll find the results of those investigations.

If the gym isn't your thing perhaps one of these "at home" gyms will fit the bill for you, go to the local gym to try them out and when you find one that you're comfortable with come back here and find the best way to get it in your home without breaking the bank.

THE BEST EQUIPMENT FOR WEIGHT LOSS.

When we're looking to lose weight exercise is just as important as a change of diet and should always be incorporated into our weight loss routine but getting the exercise isn't always as easy as going to the gym four times a week.

When we're losing weight it is essential that we burn more calories than we consume and to this end exercise equipment can become an important tool in our ongoing efforts.

Aerobic exercise, that is exercise that increases our heart rate, is the best sort of exercise for weight loss and walking or running is a good way to get this but it isn't always convenient, or safe, to walk or run around the block every day.

That's why exercise equipment can be useful, it allows us to get the right sort of exercise, at the gym or at home, in complete safety and at times that are convenient for us.

So that begs the question "What is the best type of equipment for weight loss"?

The answer to that question is that there are several options, each of which will offer us some form of effective aerobic, and therefore weight loss exercise.

Many personal trainers and weight loss exercise professionals consider four of the best equipment options for weight loss to be treadmills, ellipticals, exercise bikes, and rowing machines.

TREADMILLS.

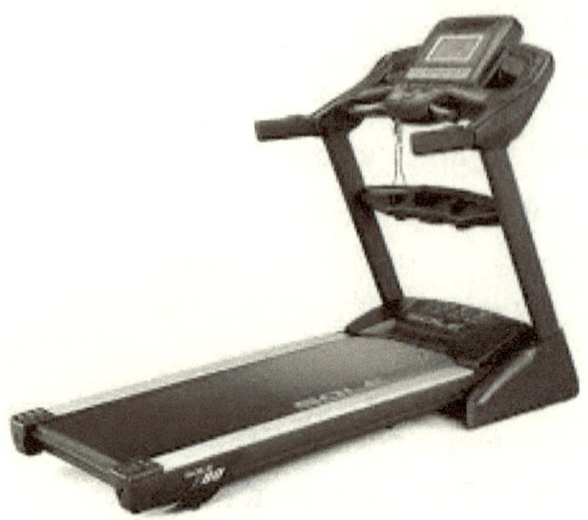

Treadmills give us the ability to go for a walk or a run, on the flat or up an incline, as fast or as slow as we need, all from the safety of our own home or the local gym.

We can purchase a treadmill almost anywhere, even on-line for as little as a few hundred dollars or as much as a few thousand dollars depending on what "extras" we would like.

A basic model will give us all the aerobic exercise we need, if we would like the bells and whistles then, of course, we must pay more for it.

If we want to own our own treadmill, before we buy it, as with the purchase of any exercise equipment, we should find somewhere that has the model we intend to buy and give it a good trial, not just once but several times over a reasonable period of time, we don't want to get our treadmill home to find after three weeks that it just isn't working for us.

There is a possible drawback to the use of a treadmill and that is that it may not be suitable for those of us who have problems with our knees or ankle joints, there is a certain amount of impact involved with the exercise.

ELLIPTICALS.

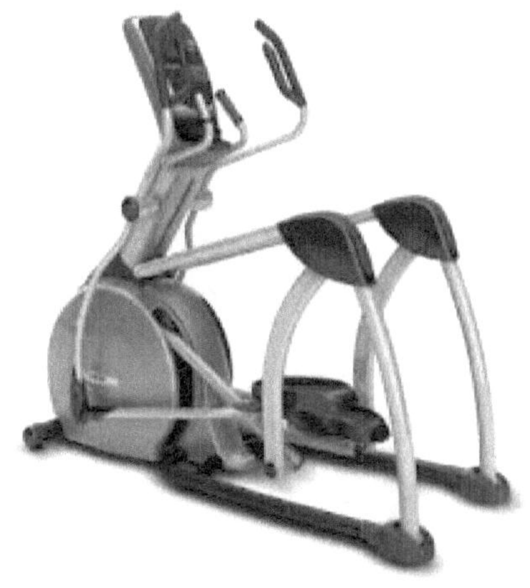

Ellipticals have all the advantages of a treadmill but without the joint jarring impact which makes an elliptical exercise machine a better choice for many of us.

We can get a good aerobic workout on an elliptical without the joint stress and many modern ellipticals have the ability to operate in reverse thereby allowing us to work a different set of muscles.

We can also find elliptical machines which have poles attached, similar to those used by skiers, to give us some upper body exercise as well.

Ellipticals are a good choice for those of us who want something a little more gentle than a treadmill but with a similar result.

EXERCISE BIKES.

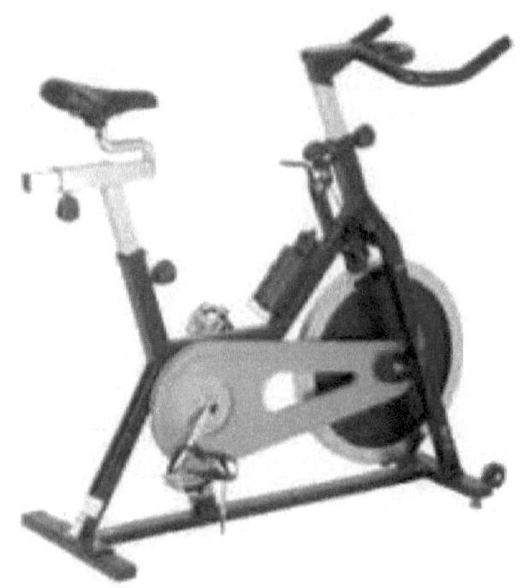

With traffic becoming so thick on many roads these days and with many motorists taking little or no care around cyclists an exercise bike is a great alternative for those of us who would prefer to cycle our way to weight loss.

Like our everyday bike our exercise bike comes in any number of different styles, each with its own advantages and disadvantages but one advantage they all have is that we can ride them in the gym or at home in front of the TV if we wish.

We can pedal away for as long as we like, drink a coffee or read a book, talk to our spouses or shout at the kids without ever leaving the saddle.

Today we can even hire or purchase an exercise bike which is just like a traditional bike or we can get one which allows us almost to lie down and pedal.

The recumbent exercise bike gives us back support while we exercise and almost all exercise bikes these days allow us to adjust the level of resistance so that we can cycle "on the flat" or "uphill" as we desire.

If you like to cycle then an exercise bike may be your answer.

ROWING MACHINES.

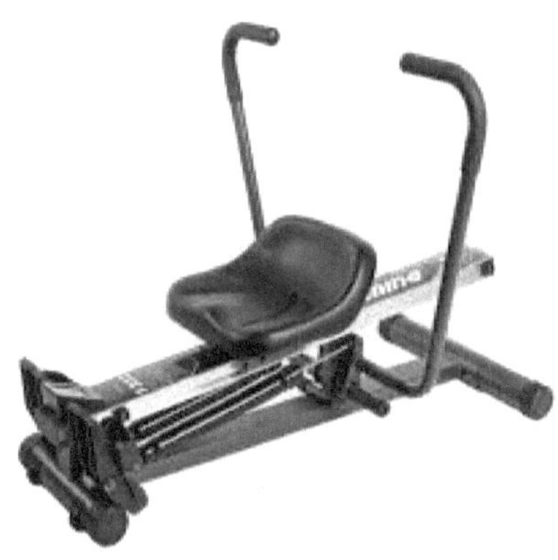

Considered by many to be the ultimate in weight loss exercise equipment, the rowing machine helps us to lose weight by exercising large groups of muscles in both our upper and lower body at the same time.

This is good for those of us who wish exercise to lose weight but are relatively time poor because with a rowing machine we can burn more calories in a shorter amount of time than with any of the other equipment we can use.

The risk of injury when using a rowing machine is also reduced because there is little or no stress or pressure on our knees and ankles.

As with all the other types of exercise equipment we can get a basic rowing machine or we can add the extras, like a fan to keep us cool as we row.

The bottom line when considering the use or purchase of exercise equipment is to try it out first to make sure that the equipment is suitable for us, that it will allow us to exercise when and where, and in a manner that suits us, after all, the best exercise equipment in the world won't do us any good if we don't use it.

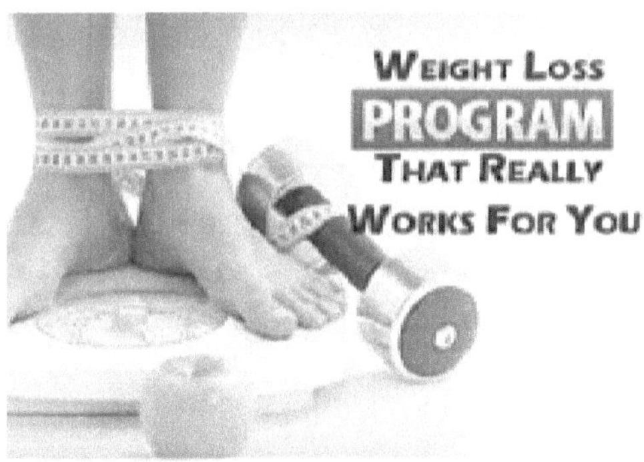

Around the world millions struggle with weight issues everyday and despite the claims that this diet or that weight loss programme will work for everyone the simple truth is that no weight loss programme will work for everybody.

We're all different, we have different lifestyles, we have different medical requirements and personalities that will require different approaches to the situation of excess weight.

However while no one thing will work for everyone something will work for everyone it's just a matter of finding the particular thing that works for you.

For some the idea of controlling their appetite is difficult, they just feel compelled to eat everything that's put in front of them and have little or no ability to say "no more thank you", some weight loss gurus attempt to approach the situation from a psychological perspective, trying to find the hidden issues which cause us to overeat, still others will tell you that you need to work yourself to exhaustion on the treadmill or remove certain foods from your diet altogether.

There are programmes around which rely on what I call "meal replacement therapy", you've seen them, instead of lunch you have a weight control shake, instead of breakfast it's a "muesli" bar.

These methods may work for some who try them but one thing is certain, they don't work on their own.

Diet pills, appetite suppressants, pre-prepared meals, hours at the gym will probably all help to some degree but they, either on their own or in combination with others may not work for you.

The trick here is to find what *will* work for you.

So how do you do that?

It's really just a matter of deciding what you can and can't do.

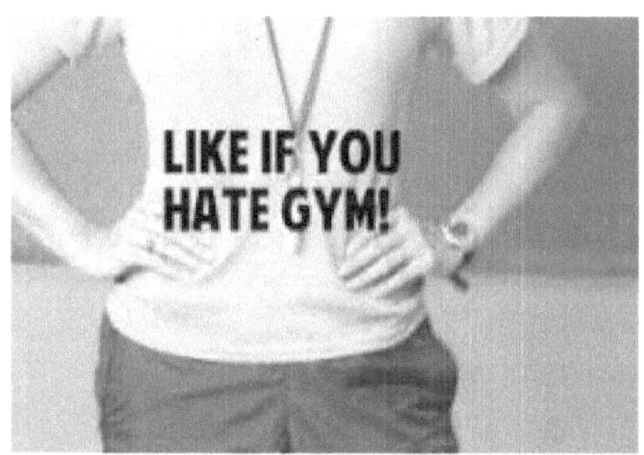

If you don't have the time or the inclination to go to the gym four times week then obviously the workout until you drop method is not for you but perhaps you might enjoy something which is energetic and fun, something like belly-dancing which is good exercise, will offer you some company while you exercise and for those who enjoy it it's fun.

Yoga might be more your speed, or good old walking, most communities these days have walking groups where you can join with others and get your gentle exercise while you have a chat about everything and nothing.

Perhaps for you it's not a lack of exercise which is the problem it might be the kind of food you eat.

We've all seen an overweight bricklayer or road worker, no-one can say that they don't get enough exercise so why do they not all look like matchsticks with the wood shaved off?

Obviously it's because they eat the wrong food, they often eat food which is heavy with fat and carbohydrates because it gives them a short term lift in their energy levels which they think is helping them do their very physical jobs and while this may be true to some extent the damage it does in terms of their weight is quite significant.

Where a lot of people go wrong when trying to formulate a weight loss programme is that they don't take into consideration their own lifestyle and personality.

It's too easy to just jump on someone else's bandwagon and follow the latest diet trends.

After all it worked for that actress who needed to lose her baby weight so it should work for me shouldn't it?

While there is nothing wrong with trying something to see if it will work your goal must be to find something which is appealing to you personally, which you can find enjoyable and something which you can stick at.

This is the most important piece of advice you will ever get when you're losing weight, find something that is appealing to you and *stick at it!*

The final piece of advice here is to have very firm and realistic goals.

"To lose weight" is not a goal it's a dream and it won't help you one bit.

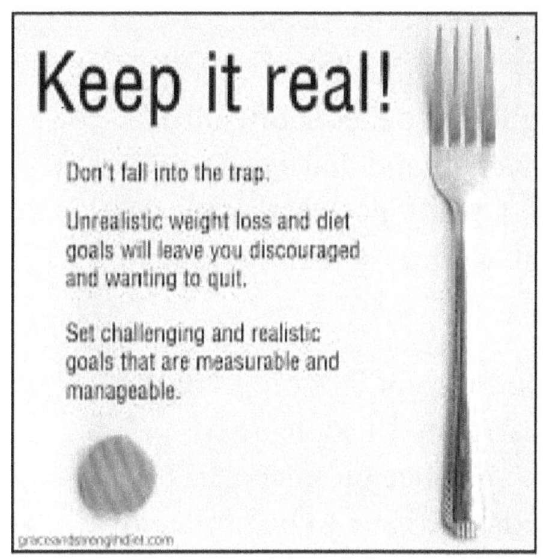

"To lose 5 kilos by July 1st" is a goal, it's measureable and it has a date on it!

Your goal must appear to you to be believable and achievable, there's no point in saying you're going to lose 10 kilos in a week if you've been struggling to lose any weight at all for some time now and you don't have to start with the big result, small goals, achieved one by one will work much better.

Remember if your attempts to lose weight make you feel unwell in any way, maybe leave you dizzy or unable to focus, stop straight away and go to see your medical professional.

Fortunately there are any number of weight loss programmes around, with a little research you're sure to find one that suits you.

THE BEST WEIGHT LOSS PROGRAMS.

When we're striving for weight loss a diet is often the first thing we turn to to lose weight and that's not a bad idea but, as with most things, a really good weight loss program, like a really good butcher, is sometimes hard to find.

For me what constitutes a good weight loss program is a one that fits quite comfortably in my lifestyle, that doesn't require any enormous sacrifice on my part, although obviously some foods etc. have to be limited or done away with altogether, one which I can afford [not all weight loss programs are cheap...] and, of course, a weight loss program that actually helps me lose weight.

In an effort to help us all find a good weight loss program that will work for each of us I've reviewed nine of the most popular weight loss programs and diets, many of which I've tried, and the results of that review is given below in no particular order.

It's as well to note that all of these will help us to lose weight, especially if we combine them a regular exercise program so it really is just a matter of finding the one that suits you best.

WEIGHT WATCHERS.

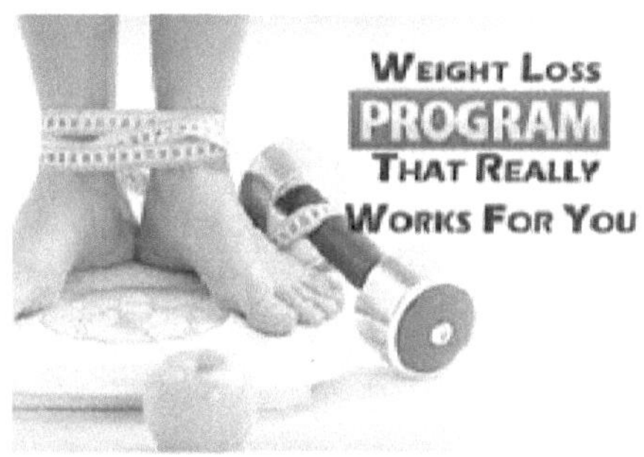

Possibly the most popular, and most successful weight loss program is the one promoted by Weight Watchers.

Weight Watchers promote the idea that losing weight is more involved that just counting calories, that a complete lifestyle overhaul is often what's needed and they're right, that's why the Weight Watchers program is so successful.

A [very] condensed overview of the Weight Watchers weight loss program goes a bit like this:

Every food is assigned a nutritional value, for example foods with higher amounts of sugar and saturated fats are assigned a higher value than those with higher amounts of protein and your food choice becomes one of foods which are nutritionally dense and light on calories as opposed to foods that are calorie heavy but nutritionally light.

The idea here is that when faced with a choice you'll learn to lean towards the food which will has more nutrients and less calories, not only because it's healthier for you but because that way you'll stay "fuller" for longer.

Couple this with the Weight Watchers support program and it has to be a good choice when we're trying to lose weight.

JENNY CRAIG WEIGHT LOSS PROGRAM.

The Jenny Craig weight loss program is also a very popular and successful weight loss regimen and it differs from that of Weight Watchers in that it promotes losing weight being as simple as restricting calorie intake and cutting down on fat and portion size and emphasizing a healthy lifestyle.

When you sign up with Jenny Craig you sign up to receive your meals pre-packaged so you'll know that the portion sizes are suitable and the food is healthy, you'll also get a personal consultant to guide you through your weight loss program from the very first day.

You get support on your weight loss journey and when you're finished with Jenny Craig you should know what a healthy balanced meal looks like and how big a portion size you should be eating.

THE BIGGEST LOSER WEIGHT LOSS PROGRAM.

Well I guess it is a weight loss program of sorts, six weeks of intense regular exercise and very healthy food is a really good way to start our weight loss efforts, not only should we lose weight but also reduce the risk of diabetes, cancer and dementia, improve the health of our hearts and boost our immune systems.

At least that's what those who believe in the biggest loser weight loss program tell us, work out hard and cut the calories and you'll be skinny in no time.

Personally I don't know if it works or not but it surely must be worth a try if you're that way inclined and let's face it, it can't do us any harm can it?

Just one word of warning, check with your doctor before you start to make sure that your body can manage the extra exercise.

HMR [HEALTH MANAGEMENT RESOURCES] MEAL REPLACEMENTS.

The idea behind the HMR weight loss program is that we can lose weight and keep it off by reducing calories [nothing new here] but it's suggested that by replacing meals with shakes and protein bars, they call them "benefit bars" and including as much suitable fruit and vegetables as we need to keep us feeling full we can lose weight without the stress of reducing our intake to the point of always feeling hungry.

Those who should know will tell us that about three times as much weight is lost, and kept off, using meal replacements as opposed to the more conventional diets and it seems to be an effective weight loss regimen especially when combined with realistic levels of regular exercise.

THE SLIM-FAST WEIGHT LOSS PROGRAM.

Similar to the HMR diet the Slim-Fast diet advocates tell us that losing weight is a simple as reducing potion sizes and thereby reducing calories.

Slim-Fast meal replacement bars, shakes and snack bars are designed to replace the first two meals of the day, that's breakfast and lunch, and also to give us something to snack on when we feel the need.

They are nutrient rich but leave room for us to eat one regular meal a day so we don't get the food withdrawal that kills so many of our weight loss efforts.

There you have it, just five reasonably good weight loss programs which should help us all to lose weight without causing us any bad side effects or dangerous health problems.

There are, of course, many more diets and weight loss programs on the market, many of which I'm sure would help us with our weight loss, as I've said above it really is just a matter of finding something that works for each of us and persisting with it until it becomes a lifestyle, then we reach the holy grail and gain that body or those health benefits we all strive for.

FIVE BAD EATING HABITS.

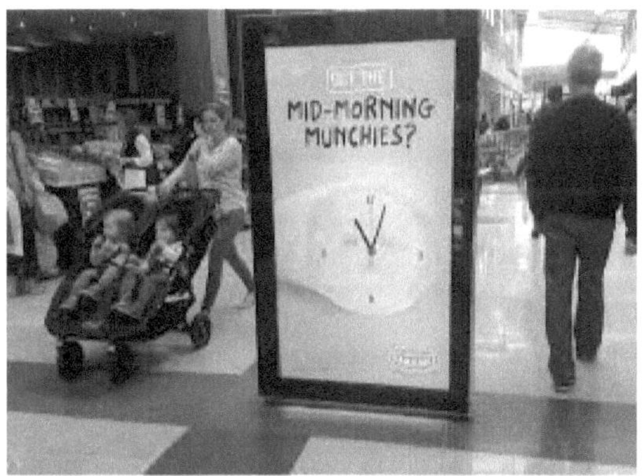

We all get hungry between meals, some more than others, but how we deal with that hunger can make all the difference to our weight loss efforts.

Personally I like to eat little and often and what I like to eat is biscuits [cookies] and other sweet, sugary snacks, and guess what.....that doesn't help me lose weight one little bit.

If, like me you just have to snack then snack on something that will satisfy your between meals hunger without ruining your diet, foods that contain high amounts of fibre, fruit, some nuts etc. is the way to go.

Leave the biscuits in the biscuit barrel and only eat them very occasionally and you'll notice the difference.

Do You Like To Eat Out?

Don't we all but dining out too often can easily lead to weight gain rather than weight loss.

Restaurants are in the business of making us want to eat more not less, that's how they make their money and they do it by adding flavour to the foods we order.

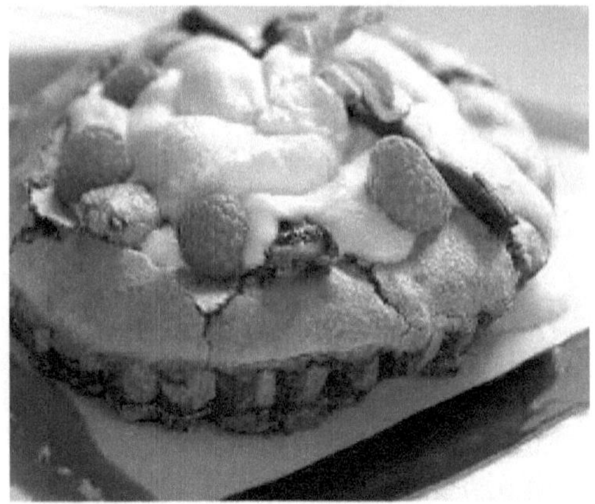

A little extra salt here, a big pinch of sugar there and cook it in butter and you've not only got a very flavoursome meal but a meal that is definitely not going to help us lose weight.

Watch the celebrity chefs on TV and you'll see what I mean.

Dine out by all means just don't do it too often.

Boredom will kill a diet in most people quicker than hunger will.

Why is that?

It's because when we're bored or uncomfortable with our situation our brain will try to correct that and how it does it is to increase the level of dopamine it produces.

Dopamine, as you may be aware, is a neurotransmitter which is responsible for our feelings of pleasure and satisfaction and one certain way to increase it is to eat!

It's a survival tactic which is built in but if we aware of it we can avoid boredom eating by pausing before we grab that biscuit or bag of potato chips or perhaps chewing some gum or doing something else to distract us from munching.

Don't get bored it can be a diet killer.

Don't Eat Rubbish For Breakfast.

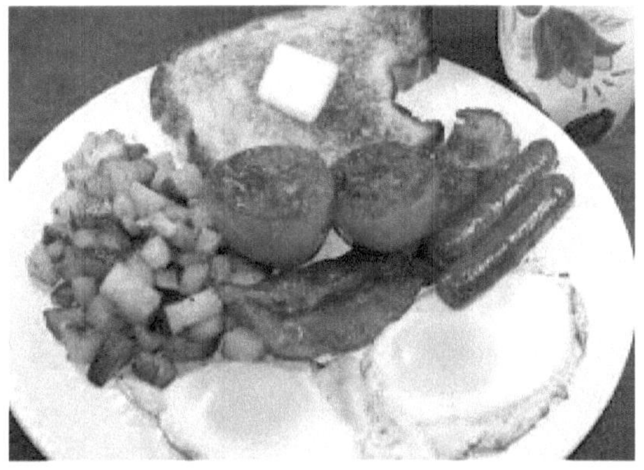

Eating a good breakfast is not only a very healthy habit to get into it's also good practice when we're determined to lose weight but what constitutes a good breakfast?

Well, while eggs make for a healthy breakfast, when we combine them with something like cheese and put them together on a bagel so that we can eat it while we're driving to work we're asking for trouble later in the day.

An egg and cheese bagel has very little fibre and a stack of carbs and calories and a breakfast like this will, after a couple of hours, lead to an energy low and the mid morning munchies.

We've all been there but there are ways to avoid the need to eat at morning tea break.

A good breakfast is essential, scrambled eggs, Greek yoghurt, oats, whole wheat cereal and the like will all do the job and we won't find ourselves at the vending machine looking for something to eat by 10.30 am.

Following on from that don't fall into the habit of missing breakfast altogether in the mistaken belief that if we miss breakfast we must obviously consume less calories.

While this is true it isn't a good idea and is certainly not a long term weight loss solution.

For years I didn't eat breakfast at all, I made all sorts of excuses, I didn't have time, I didn't like eating early in the day, I couldn't go to work on a full stomach and so on and not eating breakfast didn't help my weight problem one bit.

After I was diagnosed with type 2 diabetes and told to change my ways or risk losing a limb or worse, my eyesight, my wife insisted I eat a healthy breakfast every day and, surprise, surprise, I started to lose weight.

Since that time I've lost between 15 and 20 kilos and while I can't say that it's all as a result of eating a healthy breakfast each day it certainly has helped.

Three healthy balanced meals each day combined with sensible exercise is still the best way to lose weight.

THE BEST FOODS AND DRINKS FOR WEIGHT LOSS.

It's a well known, and scientifically proven, fact that certain foods and drinks will cause you to gain weight.

Everyone knows that if you have a diet consisting mainly of fatty, greasy or sugary food and you drink copious amounts of soft drink [soda] or alcohol you will inevitably put on weight.

Many of us have proved that in our own lives, me included, but not so many of us know that there are certain foods which will help us substantially to lose weight.

You see, when it comes to weight loss not all foods are created equal.

There are a great number of foods and drinks which will very effectively kill your appetite and increase your metabolism thereby causing you to burn more calories as you go about your daily routine.

Below I've outlined 10 of the more popular of these, try them for yourself, you may well be surprised.

COFFEE.

Surprise, surprise, coffee may not be as bad for you as it's been made out to be, especially if you're trying to lose weight.

Coffee is apparently a very healthy food, it's full of antioxidants and bioactive compounds.

[According to the NCI Dictionary of Cancer Terms a bioactive compound is a type of chemical found in small amounts in plants and certain foods (such as fruits, vegetables, nuts, oils, and whole grains). Bioactive compounds have actions in the body that may promote good health. They are being studied in the prevention of cancer, heart disease, and other diseases.

Examples of bioactive compounds include lycopene, resveratrol, lignan, tannins, and indoles.]

Coffee, as everyone knows, is chock full of caffeine, that's the reason it keeps you awake at night if you drink it before going to bed.

What most do not know however is that caffeine has been shown to up your metabolism by as much as 10 or more percent and as a consequence boost your fat burning capacity by up to almost 30 percent, indeed, according to a recent study about 4 or 5 cups of coffee per day may help you to burn an extra 150 calories.

It would seem that if you like coffee you may on a winner however your body may become tolerant to the "coffee effect" so this may, or may not, be a long term benefit.

APPLE CIDER VINEGAR.

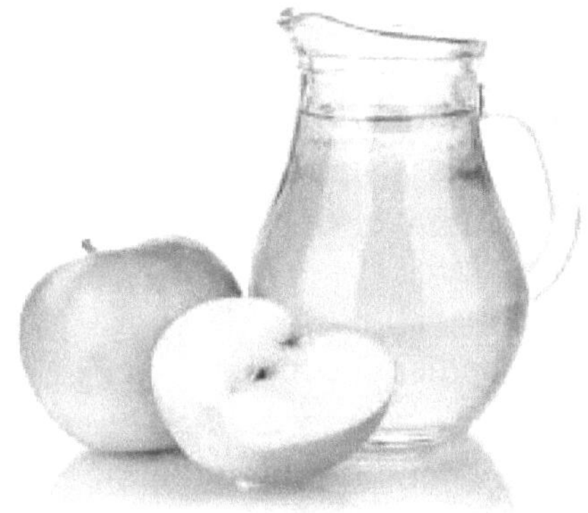

With very significant health benefits, apple cider vinegar has become extremely popular with those who subscribe to the "natural" way of looking after your health.

Apparently, if taken after a meal which is high in carbohydrates it can make a big difference to your blood sugar spike and may contribute to modest weight loss by increasing the feeling of being "full" thereby decreasing your food [and therefore your calorie] intake for the rest of your day.

One study has indicated that 1-2 tablespoons of apple cider vinegar taken daily over a period of 12 weeks produced a weight loss of about 1.5 kilogrammes.

COCONUT OIL.

Coconut oil contains fats called medium-chain triglycerides or medium-chain fatty acids and these are not the same as most other fats.

Apparently these medium-chain triglycerides are matabolised in a different way to other fatty acids and may have significantly different effects on the body.

There are studies which seem to indicate that these particular fatty acids will make you feel fuller for longer thereby reducing your calorie intake by up to 250 calories per day and boosting the number of calories you burn by up to 125 calories per day.

Other studies have focused on whether coconut oil does produce weight loss in people, the results seem to indicate that whilst weight loss was not a result of taking coconut oil a considerable reduction of waist circumference was with many reporting that taking 2 tablespoons of coconut oil per day saw their waist measurement reduce.

Those of us who struggle with "belly fat" may well be advised to try it!

NUTS.

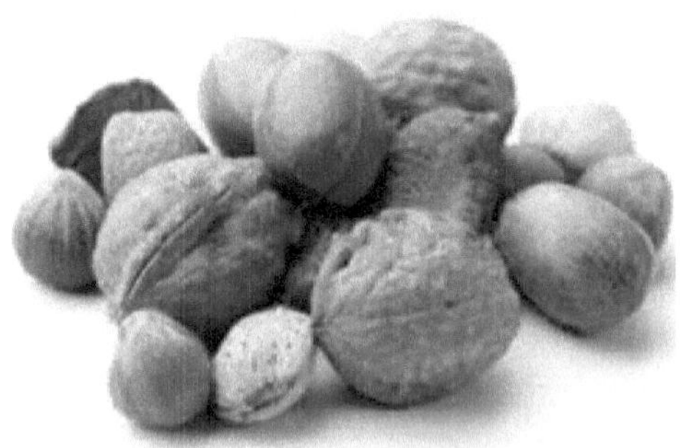

Surprising as it may seem, and although nuts are very high in fat, they are amongst the best foods on the planet when it comes to helping us lose weight.

Nuts are high in fibre, protein and the healthy type fats as well as having few carbohydrates and because of the way nuts are built the carbs which they do have are very hard for the body to absorb.

Apparently about 15 percent of the carbs in nuts don't ever get absorbed, they just pass straight through.

Nuts are also very satisfying, they make you feel full without all the nasties and there is even some evidence that they help to boost your metabolism, giving you more energy to burn even more calories.

In one recent controlled study it was shown that people who regularly eat nuts tend to weigh less and controlled trials have shown a significant reduction in waist size.

It has been proven time and again that nuts in general and peanuts in particular are some of the best weight loss foods we can eat, they easily fill us up, they may increase our metabolism and a greater part of the calories they contain is wasted.

LEAN MEAT AND FISH.

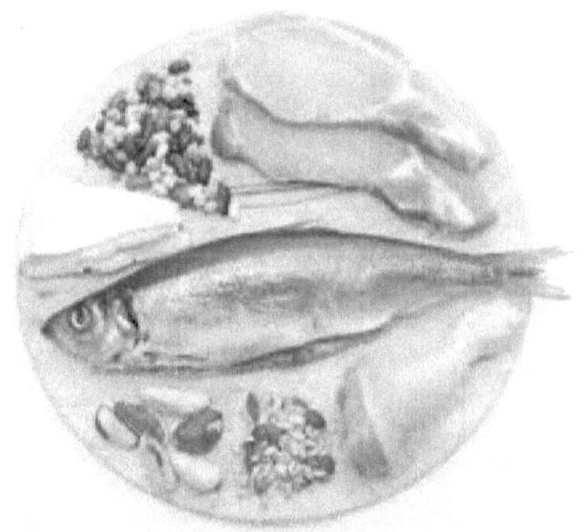

Good protein and plenty of it may well be your best friend when it comes to losing those extra kilos and it's well known that most fish and lean meat are the best sources of the best protein.

A number of reliable studies indicate that a diet which includes reasonable quantities of good quality protein may up your metabolism and help to burn an extra 100 to 250 calories every day.

A high protein diet may also help to curb those late night raids on the refrigerator and help prevent any regaining of weight during your stable periods.

Getting enough good protein in your diet isn't always easy so I would recommend you get yourself something like a Cron-o-meter [at the time of writing they're about $3 from Amazon] to help you keep track and make sure you're getting all the protein you need.

As I said above, lean meat and fish are some of the best sources of good protein and good protein may well be you answer to weight loss.

GREEN TEA.

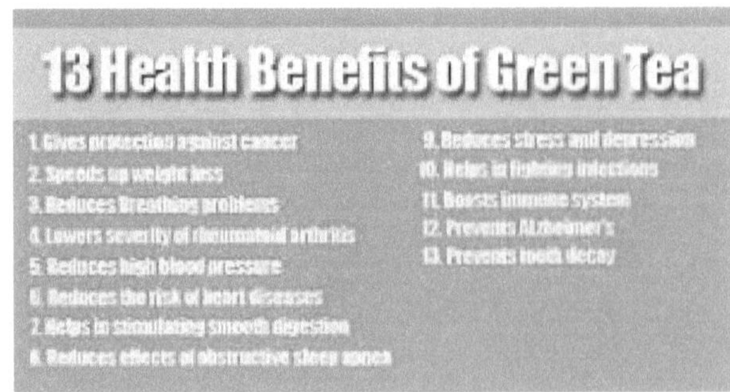

If you don't like coffee you might consider replacing it with green tea which is another beverage which will help with your weight loss.

Green tea, like coffee, does have certain amounts of caffeine to boost your metabolism but green tea also contains several other bioactive compounds including an antioxidant called EGCG which seems to be very beneficial, not only for weight loss but also for brain health, heart health and as a possible cancer preventative. [Please don't rely on this as a treatment for cancer, medical advice is always the best path to follow.]

The evidence is not conclusive however the consumption of green tea has been shown to aid in weight loss and especially in the loss of "belly fat".

BOILED POTATOES.

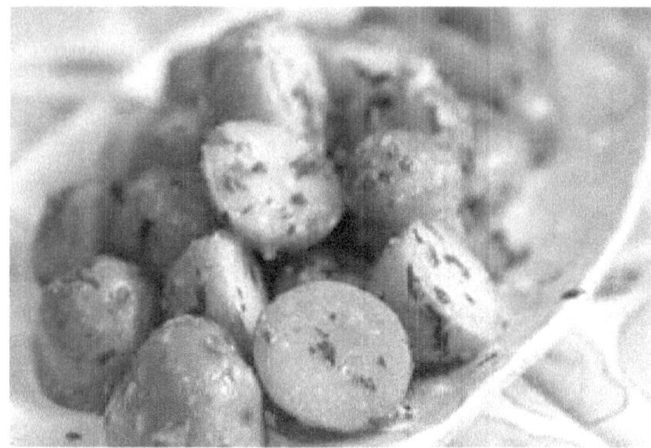

Potatoes, or "spuds" as I call them, can be both a blessing and a curse in your fight to lose weight depending on what you do with them once they're peeled.

As french fries or chips, cooked in a deep fryer and soaked in fat, they'll make you put on weight faster than almost anything else but whole potatoes, boiled or baked are a different story.

The "fullness factor", as measured by the satiety index, indicates that white boiled potatoes are the very best thing you can eat to make you feel "full" and thereby cause you to eat less at each meal.

If you fill up on spuds there's no room for more fattening food.

Of course you shouldn't try to live on just white boiled potatoes, you would soon find yourself lacking in other essential nutrients, but as part of your weight loss strategy it may well be a good idea to include perhaps an extra helping of boiled spuds, without, of course, the added butter we all love to put in our mash.

If you wanted to take the weight loss benefits of potatoes to the next level just cool them before you eat them.

Cooling apparently increases the amount of resistant starch which is a fibre-like substance that may also help you to lose weight.

CHILLI PEPPERS.

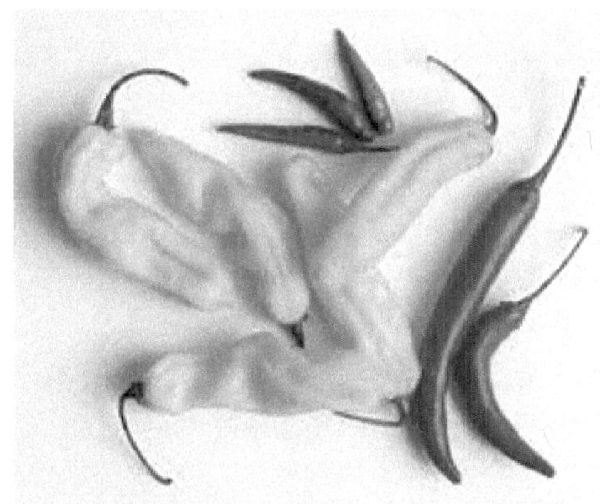

Almost all, if not all, hot peppers contain a substance called capsaicin which has been proven in many studies to reduce the appetite and boost the metabolism.

It is for this reason that a great majority of weight loss supplements you can purchase over the counter contain certain amounts of capsaicin and if you like a little spice in your food then eating more chilli may well be a good thing for your weight loss efforts.

That said it doesn't hold good for people who eat spicy food on a regular basis indicating that a tolerance to hot spices may build up over time.

WHOLE EGG.

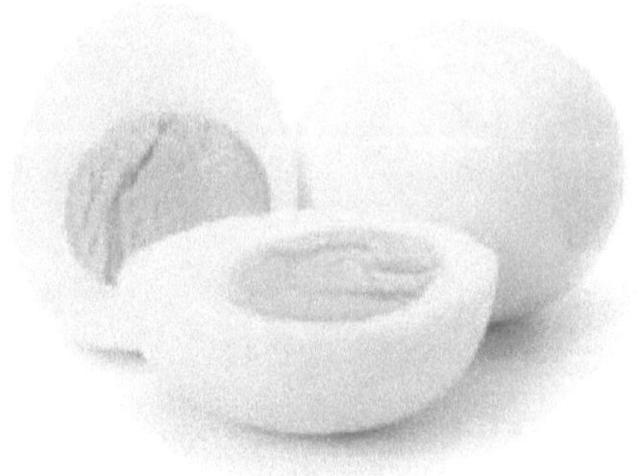

Is whole egg a wonder food or do we leave it alone?

Over the years eggs have been blamed for causing high cholesterol in those who consumed them but recent studies have shown that eggs generally have very little or no effect on the cholesterol levels of those who eat them.

Many well respected studies have shown that eating eggs for breakfast can be very beneficial when trying to lose weight.

Eggs make you feel more full and those who ate eggs instead of, for example, bagels for breakfast ended up eating less for the next 36 hours.

That's an impressive statistic and yet another study has shown that eggs for breakfast were the reason for a 65% greater weight loss in those who ate them when compared to those who ate bagels even though both contain the same number of calories.

If you're intolerant of eggs don't fret any breakfast which is protein rich and full of nutrients should work just as well.

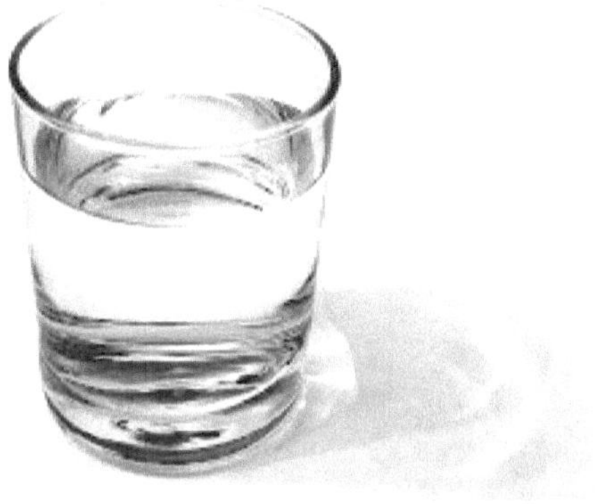

Water, we've been told ever since we were children that drinking water is good for us and indeed it is but how many of us who struggle with our weight realise that drinking water has a surprising weight loss effect.

Drinking half a litre [500cc] of water can increase your metabolism by as much as 30% for 90 minutes especially if you drink it cold because your body has to use energy to warm the water to body temperature once you've consumed it.

Also, drinking the same half a litre of water before meals will increase your feeling of fullness thereby causing you to eat less.

What all of this proves is that instead of starving yourself in order to lose weight if you change your diet and eat the right foods and drink the right beverages you can almost put your weight loss on "autopilot" and enjoy meal times again.

FOOD ADDICTION.

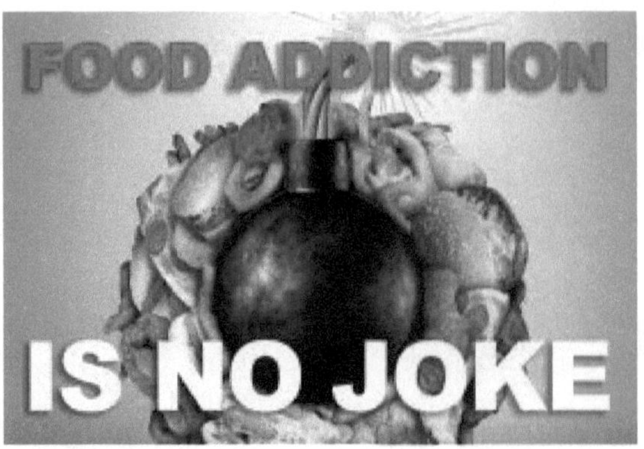

Everyone will overdose on unhealthy food every once in a while but could they be considered as food addicts?

Probably not.

It's when you have food cravings that you are unable to control that you need to take a serious look at the possibility that you may indeed be a food addict.

Many learned people in the medical field consider that food addiction is just as real, and just as potentially fatal as addiction to cigarettes or hard drugs.

So how do you tell if you're a food addict?

Again, medical opinion says that if you have an uncontrollable craving for a particular food or types of food and if, when you are unable to get your "fix" you have withdrawal symptoms like depression, nausea and

headaches, then the probability is that you are in fact
food addicted.

Food addicts get comfort from particular foods, they may
engage in binge eating and their food cravings can be
both psychological and physical.

Also it would seem that there are different types of food
addiction.

Uncontrollable over-eating, where someone will binge on
food, [pig out we used to call it] in sessions that can last
for several days, eat when they're not hungry, scoff their
food or eat it very quickly, perhaps even furtively, is one
form of food addiction.

Another is bulimia which is defined in the Cambridge
dictionary as "a mental illness in which someone eats in
an uncontrolled way and in large amounts, and
then vomits intentionally".

Deliberately over-eating and then purging your system
by vomiting or taking laxatives or something similar is
definitely a form of food addiction.

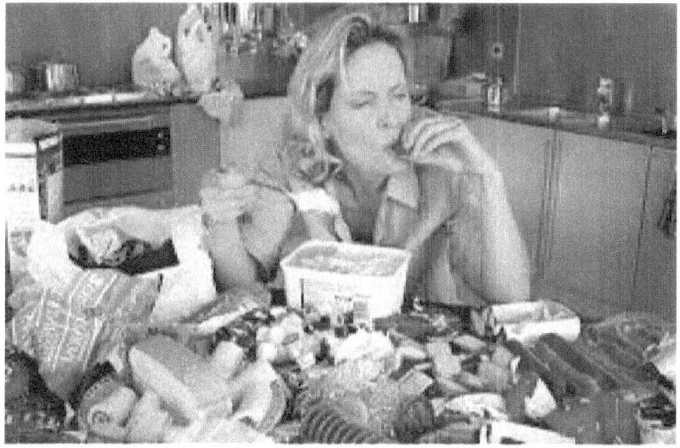

Some of the tell-tale signs here are eating alone, consuming enormous amounts of food in one go and being preoccupied with your weight.

On the other side of the same coin is anorexia.

Anorexia gets its fair share of publicity and we've all seen someone who suffers from this unfortunate condition, most look like walking skeletons.

Anorexics will attempt to starve themselves in order to attain what they consider to be their goal weight.

Medically, anorexics tend to be, on average, about 20% below the normal body weight for someone of a similar height and build and most have a phobia about the consumption of food.

Those suffering from anorexia normally are uncomfortable eating in the presence of others, most are almost paranoid about not putting on weight, they tend to have certain rituals when it comes to eating and may suffer from depression as a result.

These are all forms of food addiction in one way or another and I'm sure there are more forms of food addiction than I've mentioned here, the good news is that food addiction in all its forms is very treatable.

A variety of measures may be taken to combat or cure food addiction.

These include consulting with a psychotherapist to work out new ways to deal with the underlying issues which cause the food addiction in the first place, the therapist can help to identify these issues and develop a plan to overcome the problem.

Often the food addicts will adopt a similar approach to their situation as does an alcoholic to his.

For instance this may involve first if all admitting that they have a problem, stating their desire to, and belief that they can, break the hold which food has over their lives and so on.

Support groups and friends/family can be important sources of strength and just being aware that they are not alone in their struggle is often very beneficial.

There is no scientific evidence at this point to suggest that food addiction is a genetically-based illness there is, however, reason to believe that eating habits are passed from parents to children, how often do you see an overweight child walking beside and overweight parent?

With this in mind many food addicts only look for help when they realise that their illness may affect the lives of their offspring.

No one at this point really knows if food addiction can ever be permanently cured but it certainly can be treated, food addicts can be helped in much the same way as alcoholics are helped and food addicts should never lose sight of that fact.

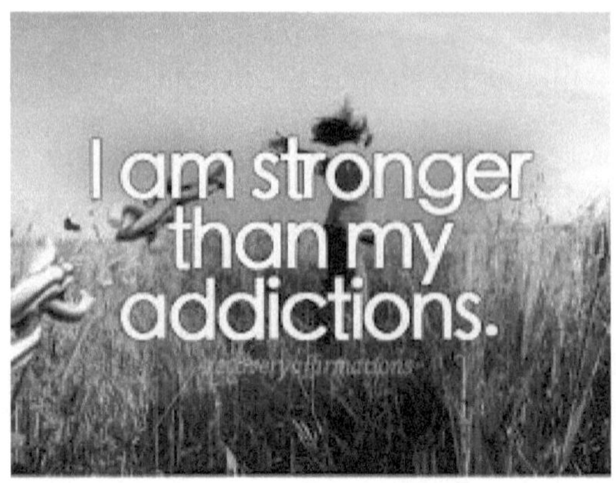

Given time the food addict can learn to make healthier, better informed food choices which will, with patience and persistence, give them the ability to keep their weight under control.

Beating food addiction is never going to be easy but with some [professional] help it can be done and the rewards in terms of better health, more self esteem and the knowledge that their children will not be likewise affected should be all the incentive needed to win the battle.

HOW DO YOU EAT?

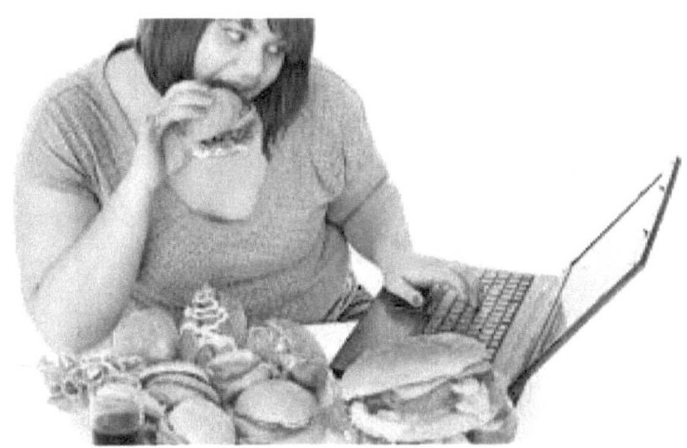

Stupid question, after all eating comes as naturally to us all as breathing doesn't it?

However the question remains and, believe it or not, the way you consume your food may be having a significant impact on your quest to lose weight.

If you've never been taught, or learned, to eat properly then you may never be able to successfully diet to lose weight.

I'm not talking here about your table manners, etiquette etc. because in terms of you losing weight these things are irrelevant, however your eating *habits* are relevant and important and by correcting any inappropriate eating habits you may find yourself losing weight without really trying too hard.

First things first, most of us today live in a hurried world where the pace of life has only two speeds, fast or faster.

We rush here and there, we have to get the children to school on time, we can't be late for work, mustn't miss the train and so on.

This rush inevitably spills over into our eating habits.

We rush our meals, eat on the go and rarely, if ever, take the time to sit down and eat slowly.

Taking your time over a good meal, eating slowly and chewing food properly is one of the least experienced but most pleasurable things you can do for yourself.

Any number of scientific studies have shown that the brain runs about ten minutes behind the mouth when it comes to the stomach feeling full.

This means that we continue to eat when, in fact, we have had enough and our stomachs don't need or want any more food.

Most of us have, at some time in our lives, left the dinner table and immediately wished we hadn't eaten so much.

Each meal, regardless of whether it's breakfast lunch or dinner, should be enjoyed at a leisurely pace.

If we have company then good conversation can slow your eating, resting your fork before putting more food on it and never gathering food onto your fork before you've finished the food you already have in your mouth will all help to slow the pace of your eating and will give you the added benefit of much better digestion at the same time.

Chewing your food slowly and thoroughly and drinking plenty of water between courses will also help.

Just as importantly, wait ten minutes after you finish your main course before you order dessert, you may well find that you don't have room for it regardless of how enticing it is.

If you're eating at home place your food containers, saucepans, serving dishes etc. away from the table so that you have to get up from your seat to get more food.

Often you just won't!

Another tip is to put your snacks into a dish or onto a plate instead of eating them directly from the box.

It's very easy to eat too much without thinking when the full box of potato chips is right next to you on the lounge.

The same goes for eating while you're doing something else.

If you snack while you watch TV for example there's a good chance you'll eat too much, most of us will do it without thinking.

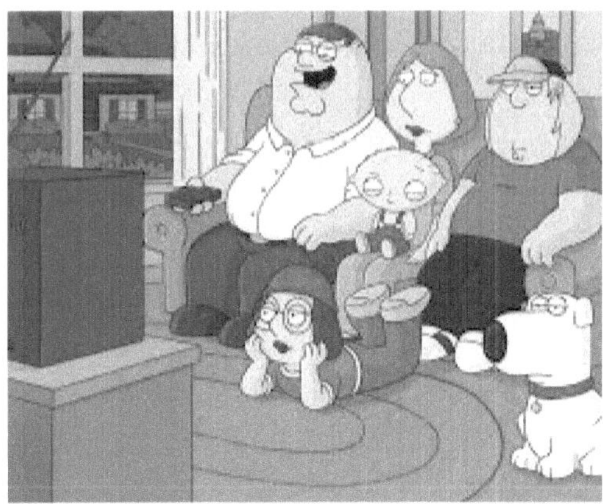

Only eating at the table is a very good habit to get into when you're losing weight, eating elsewhere could easily lead you to eat too much.

Another bad idea, one which many of us are taught as children, is that we should eat all the food on our plate.

If you're eating out, at a friend's for example, and you like to be polite and not offend your host just ask them not to overfill your plate, no-one will take offense at being asked to help you with something like that.

Don't feel that you have to eat the food just because it's there, explain to your host that rather than not liking the food you simply cannot put all that food into your stomach.

It's easier than it sounds and you'll be the healthier for it.

Another way to help you to "eat right" is not to keep any food in plain sight.

If the food or the snacks are where you can see them they become a temptation which is often difficult to resist.

Keep all of your food and snacks in the refrigerator or the pantry, out of sight is indeed out of mind and is very helpful when it comes to losing weight.

Now we're all human and you're no different to the rest of us, there will undoubtedly be times when you give in to the temptation to have an extra serving of that delicious dessert or eat that whole bar of chocolate, it's important that you don't make yourself feel bad about it.

Accept that you're human and get back to your correct way of eating, scolding yourself for a mistake will only make matters worse and then you may well start eating out of frustration and give up entirely.

It's much better to lose one day of your weight loss programme than to give up altogether.

One final thought, rarely do worthwhile results come without effort and sacrifice and that is especially true when we're talking about weight loss, depending on the person you are your journey to a better, slimmer, healthier you may take a great deal of conscious effort and not a little sacrifice but with willpower and the help of those who love you a healthier, slimmer you will be the end result of your endeavours.

HOW TO LOSE WEIGHT FAST.

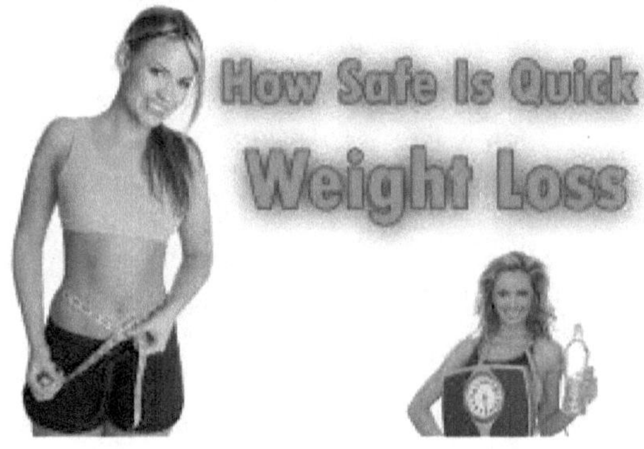

Fast weight loss is generally not a good idea as it can cause all kinds of other health problems however if we have a genuine reason to lose weight fast, we're getting married for example and we obviously want to look our best, then here are some tips to help us lose weight fast in a healthy way.

1. Eat breakfast.

When we miss breakfast rather than helping us to lose weight [by not consuming so many calories] it actually has the opposite effect.

When we don't eat breakfast our metabolism has trouble getting started for the day and as a consequence the body's natural response is to increase its insulin production. What happens then is the next time we eat we get a huge spike in our blood sugar levels which in turn leaves us feeling hungry shortly afterwards.

The smart answer is to force ourselves to eat something for breakfast, it doesn't have to be much but it does need to be healthy, scrambled egg on toast, a yoghurt smoothie, a small bowl of oats or something similar will do it.

2. Drink Water.

We should all know that drinking water is good for our health, it helps with digestion, it flushes out all the nasties from our system, prevents dehydration and so on but how many of us are aware that drinking a glass or two of the wet stuff 30 minutes or so before we eat will help with our weight loss?

The water will give us a feeling of being less hungry and we will therefore eat less, making it that much easier to lose weight.

3. More Fruit and Veg.

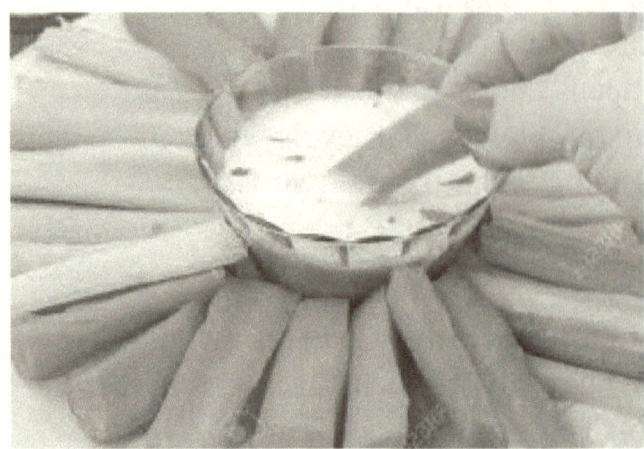

We should concentrate on trying to eat more fruit and vegetables rather than eating less carbs and fat.

The theory here is that it will be easier for us to get all the fibre and all the nutrients we need without the feeling we get from being deprived of part of our normal diet and we'll be more satisfied for longer.

4. Less sugar.

One easy way to get more fruit is to eat fruit for dessert instead of those sugar laden ice creams or puddings we so love.

Frozen mashed bananas or frozen grapes make a very tasty substitute for ice cream and a pear or apple zapped in the microwave for a minute or two and spinkled with cinnamon makes a great, and guilt free dessert.

5. Slow Down When We Eat.

We've all done it, gulped our food down when we're in a hurry or we're distracted by something more important.

It takes a little bit of time for our stomach to tell our brain it's full, until that message reaches the control centre our natural tendency is to just keep eating.

By the time the message gets through we're over full, sometimes to the point of feeling a little, well, stuffed.

The answer is to slow down when we're eating, take our time and give ourselves the opportunity to stop before we eat too much.

Before we go for that extra helping of dessert we should ask ourselves if we're really still hungry or do we just like it a little too much.

6. Give sweet drinks the shove.

We all like a glass of soda now and again and many of us, myself included, put a little extra sugar in our coffee to sweeten it up a bit but if we can give the sweet sugary drinks away we'll notice a measurable difference in a very short time.

Sugary drinks do very little for us in terms of our weight or our health and we'll all be much healthier, and slimmer, if we just don't drink them or at least cut down our intake as much as we can.

7. Same deal with the salty snacks.

Potato chips, pretzels and the like all contain a high degree of salt which causes us to retain water which in turn makes us bloat up.

Instead of munching on the salty snacks try a carrot stick or some celery, dip it in some healthy guacamole or something similar and you'll not only feel fuller for longer you'll be doing your fast weight loss efforts a favour as well.

8. Don't eat a big dinner.

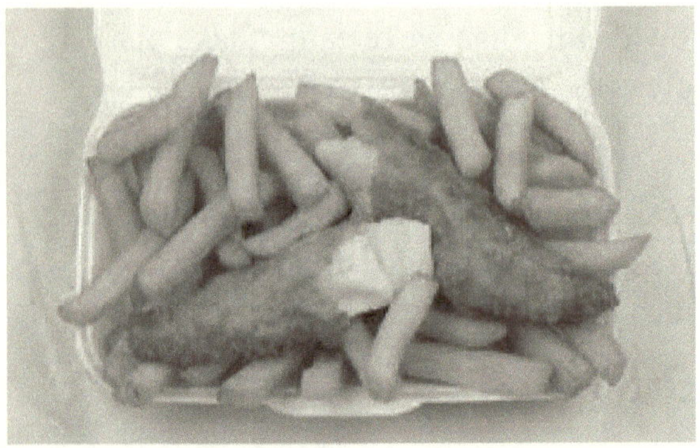

Before you get upset at this idea I'm not suggesting that we don't eat as much food as we need but just that we shouldn't eat it in the evening.

Our bodies digest food at different rates depending on the time of our day that we eat.

The norm in modern society is to eat little or no breakfast, not much more for lunch and nearly our entire food intake we have at night.

The science tells us that food consumed at night is not digested nearly as well as that eaten earlier in the day so the suggestion here is that we reverse, as best we can, the times we eat our meals, the biggest meal should be breakfast then lunch with just a small portion for dinner in the evening.

Of course the time we eat will always be relevant to "our" day; if you're a shift worker for example you must eat according to your own "day".

9. Get regular exercise.

It is, unfortunately, a fact of life that losing weight, fast or otherwise, is much more difficult if we don't get regular exercise and not just "exercise" but the right kind of exercise.

Going to the gym once a week for an hour just isn't going to do it even if we work our butts off for that hour.

We must find an exercise program that will work for us, and we're all different in that respect, and then we must stick to it.

Write it into our calendar, make our exercise an appointment we must keep just like a visit to the doctor or an appointment with our accountant and don't default on that.

It really is easy to find something else to do instead of doing our daily sit-ups but if we're serious about trimming down and losing weight quickly then this is a must do so, as Nike not so subtly put it, "just do it!"

10. Focus on small goals.

Last but by no means least we must program ourselves to focus on small goals.

We should set ourselves a target when we begin our weight loss program but most of us will set the bar way too high, especially if it's fast weight loss we're after, and it then becomes too easy to give up when we find we can't reach the goals we've set.

There's nothing wrong with reaching for the stars but every journey into outer space begins with a trip to the moon and so it must be when we begin our weight loss journey.

When we see ourselves reaching the modest goals we've set for ourselves it gives us the encouragement we need to strive for the next goal, to take the next step, to lose the next few kilos and when we achieve that goal we move on again, over a period of time we can look back and see just how far we've come in terms of our weight loss and, take my word for this, we'll feel incredible, we'll look in the mirror and say "wow" look what I've achieved, look how much weight I've lost, how good do I look now!

PS Don't forget, the "fast" in fast weight loss is a relative term, what is fast for me may not be fast for you so you must decide just how fast and how far you want to go but most of all, don't give up and..... enjoy.

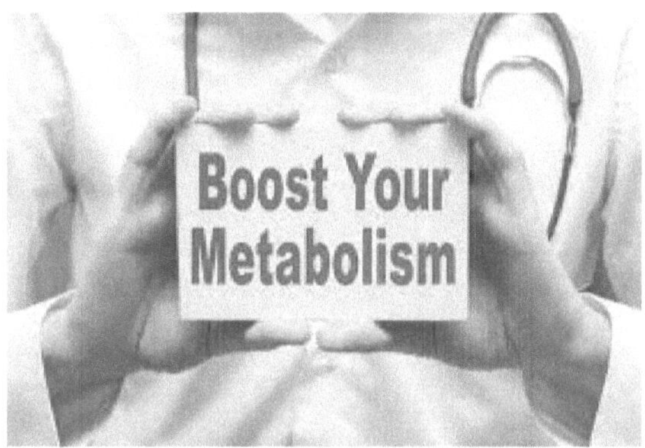

We all know that if we can increase our metabolism we are more likely to lose weight but what actually is "metabolism" and why does it concern us?

Metabolism is the process our bodies use to convert the food and drink we consume into energy and the more energy we have the faster we burn the calories we consume every day.

A "faster" metabolism might seem like the holy grail of weight loss, a bit like a wallet that refills itself whenever the money is running low but it is possible for each of us, young or old[er], fit or not so fit, to increase our metabolism.

As we get older it's natural for our mctabolism to slow down, it's just like getting wrinkles, but, just as we can, if we so choose, get Botox to smooth out those unwelcome wrinkles there are things we can do, many of them free, to help boost our metabolism.

Possibly the easiest is definitely free, that is to get some early morning sunlight!

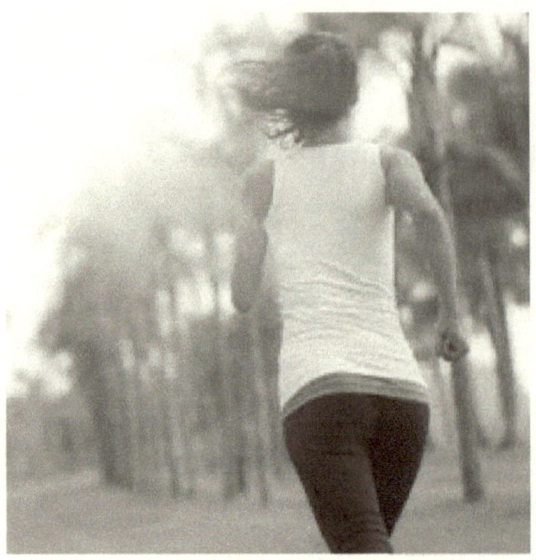

Scientific research at Northwestern University's Feinberg School of Medicine has shown that, independent of other factors relating to metabolism like age, exercise or calorie intake, those who rise early and get the early morning sun have a lower body mass index than those who get the majority of their sunlight later in the day.

Another way to boost our metabolism is to get into some serious exercise.

Building our muscle strength has been shown to significantly increase our resting metabolic rate over those of us who have a greater proportion of fat on our bodies, when we exercise we therefore get a double whammy of benefit!

Our diet can also have a very beneficial effect on our metabolism.

Green tea, for example, is a great metabolism booster, the combination of caffeine and antioxidants which are both in green tea will increase our metabolism, just a few sips a few times a day will do wonders.

Putting extra fibre on our daily menu will also boost our metabolism as well as help control our appetites by keeping us fuller for longer.

The American Journal of Clinical Nutrition recently published research which indicates that those of us who have high fibre diets burn about 100 calories a day more that those who don't.

If, like me you enjoy food with a bit of spice then you're already on your way to a higher metabolism.

Research from a number of institutions has shown that consuming food with a small amount of capsaicin has the effect of increasing the amount of calories we burn without affecting our blood pressure, thus making it a relatively safe way to go for those of us who, by reason of other health conditions, can't undertake too much high energy exercise.

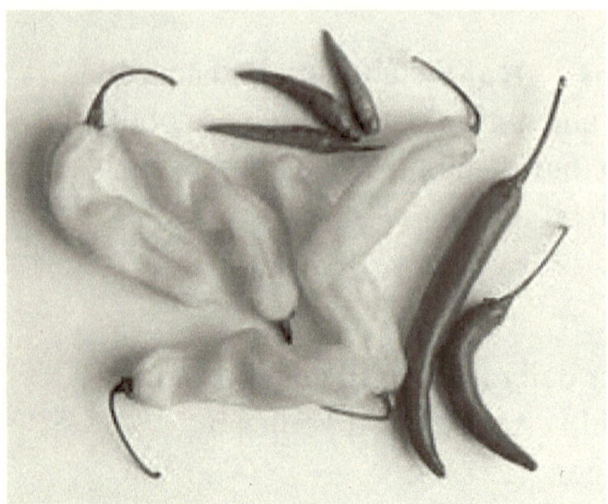

Capsaicin is the spice that gives chillies their "wonderful" heat but even if we can't stomach chillies just adding some paprika to our meals will do the job.

A good night's sleep also plays a part in boosting our metabolism with the boffins at the University of São Paulo in Brazil finding a link between melatonin, the sleep hormone, and leptin, a hormone which helps to tell our stomachs that they're full and satisfied.

A good night's sleep will apparently help us to avoid unhealthy snacks during the day and this in turn will prevent the slowing down of our metabolism which is one of the results of those sugary, fatty snacks.

Obviously a good night's sleep also has many other benefits apart from those associated with our metabolic rate which makes it a really good idea.

We've been told, too many times to count, that a big glass of water before a meal is a good idea when we're trying to lose weight, it make us feel full and so we're inclined to eat less but what we've rarely, if ever, been told is that a glass of cold water before a meal will also boost our metabolism.

Scientific studies reported in the Journal of Endocrinology & Metabolism tell us that drinking cold water increases our metabolic rate by as much as 4.5% so drinking a glass of cold water before a meal doubles the weight loss benefit, must be worth a try!!!

MORE WAYS TO BOOST YOUR METABOLISM.

In the previous chapter I discussed seven ways we can all boost our metabolism, today I have another six metabolism boosting ideas which we can all use to our advantage when we're losing weight.

Drinking more coffee may sound like something we'd all be happy to do and the research coming out of King's College in London has shown that just by adding about 100 grams of caffeine to our daily intake, [that's just one cup of coffee], may boost our metabolism to the degree that we burn an extra 150 calories.

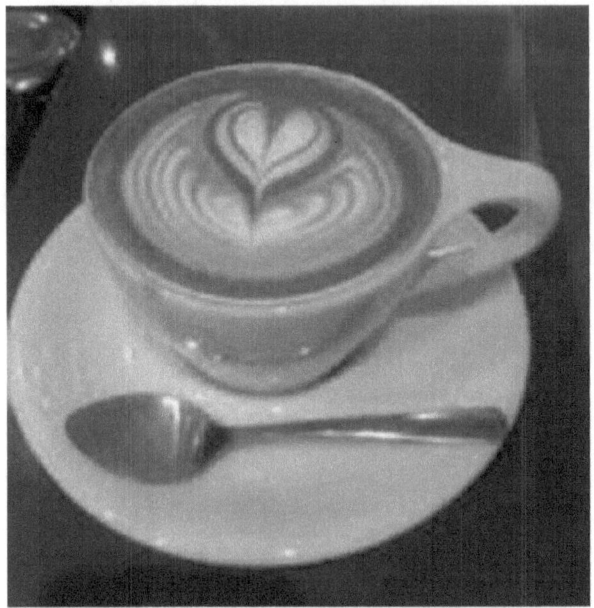

Now 150 calories per day may not seem like much in the overall scheme of things but that 150 extra calories we burn each day could add up to a weight loss of up to 1/2 a kilo [that's about 1.1/2 pounds] each month.

Fermented vegetables such as sauerkraut and pickles are not to everyone's taste but they are undeniably good for us in so many ways not the least of which is in their ability to boost our metabolism.

Researchers at Imperial College London have discovered a link between the ingestion of the probiotics found in such fermented foods and a boost in metabolism together with a decrease in our bodies ability to absorb and store fat.

By adding sauerkraut or pickles or yoghurt and the like to our meals we are not only increasing our consumption of probiotics, which has to be a good thing, but also boosting our metabolism and thereby helping with our weight loss.

Another easy way to increase our metabolism is to turn off the heat and crank up the air-conditioner at home.

The Journal of Clinical Investigation has reliably reported that if we keep the temperature at home to around 60 degrees Fahrenheit [that's about 16 degrees Celsius] for 10 days we will significantly increase our levels of healthy brown adipose tissue.

Why should that matter?

It seems that healthy brown adipose tissue has the ability to increase our metabolism and burn off any dangerous visceral fat we may have.

Again a double benefit, not only do we boost our metabolism but we save on our heating bills!

Do you visit the gym or do you prefer to get your exercise at home?

It really doesn't matter, what does matter, for the purpose of boosting our metabolism, is that we up the intensity of our workouts a couple of times a week.

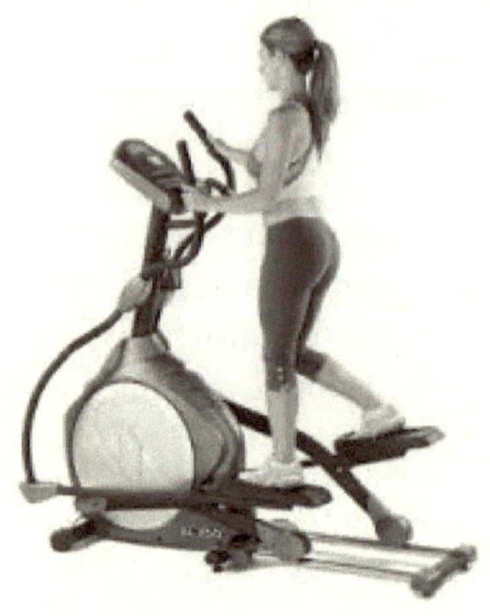

Those smart people at the University of New South Wales in Australia have discovered that if we add some very high intensity interval training twice a week it will not only lead to us losing significant body fat but it will also boost our metabolic rate for about 72 hours after we leave the shower when we're finished.

And how about that thing that's been almost welded to our ears for the past how many years?

It seems that one of the best things we can do, not only for our brain but also for our body is to just cool it and leave the mobile [cell] phone on the kitchen bench once in a while.

According to researchers at the National Institute on Drug Abuse it takes less than an hour a day of mobile phone use to affect the glucose metabolism in our brain and those at Northwestern University have found that the blue light which is emitted from those phones [and likewise our computers] have an negative impact on our circadian rhythms which makes it more difficult for us to get the right amount of sleep which, in turn, slows our metabolism.

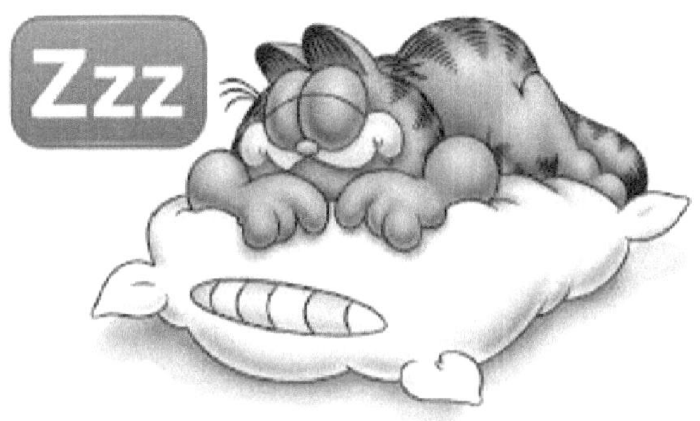

[If you don't know, according to the National Sleep Foundation "Your circadian rhythm is basically a 24-hour internal clock that is running in the background of your brain and cycles between sleepiness and alertness at regular intervals. It's also known as your sleep/wake cycle."]

Last but by no means least for this chapter on ways to boost our metabolism we must consider stress.

Many believe that a high stress level is good for their productivity but staying stressed may be compromising our metabolism.

When we get stressed our bodies produce more of the hormone cortisol which is the hormone which triggers the accumulation of belly fat.

A number of studies over the years have linked high cortisol levels with a slow metabolism, increasing our risk of obesity and making it essential for our weight loss efforts for us to slow down and de-stress when we can.

A lack of stress in our lives has also been shown to contribute to the achievement of our weight loss goals and the maintenance of that weight loss.

If we have some stubborn weight we can't seem to move it may well be worth taking an extended break from as much stress as we can, slowing down and relaxing might be just as important in the end as hitting the gym and working our butts off in the effort to boost our metabolism.

Many of us have been conditioned over many years to eat at certain times of the day and we do so with no regard to how hungry we are at the time.

When we were young many of our parents insisted we sit down for breakfast at the beginning of the day and that's an excellent idea, then we were made to eat lunch in the middle of the day and dinner was on the table at six o'clock when dad got home from work.

Often, from a very early age we were given a snack between breakfast and lunch and perhaps, as we got older, another snack when we arrived home from school.

Even supper before bed is somewhat of an institution in many households.

I'm not surprised so many of us struggle with weight issues!

And it's not just young people who live with this kind of routine, as we grow older it often becomes entrenched in our way of life.

I know that for many years I had to have supper during the evening and it, more often than not, consisted of something very sweet or very fattening.

I'd go to bed on a full stomach and have no chance of burning off those calories during the night.

No wonder I ended up a jelly ball!

If this is you, like me you must seek out a way to change your eating habits and, as with any other thing we do habitually in our lives, it isn't easy.

The first thing to understand is that we should only eat when we're actually hungry.

It may seem an obvious thing to say but when I looked at my own eating habits I realised that I would go to the fridge when I was bored, I'd eat a whole big packet of potato chips when I was on a long drive, when something made me sad I would find some solace in a snack of something or other and, more often than not, as I said above, it would be something very sweet or very fattening.

Changing habits like these isn't easy but it can be done, as I've proved in my own life, with just a little persistence and some determination.

If you like to snack that's fine just do so with healthy alternatives.

Now I'm not a fruit lover, I don't eat apples or oranges and I don't drink copious amounts of water so, for me, finding a way to overcome the bad snacking habits of a lifetime was something of a challenge.

You may find yourself in the same situation and I must tell you persistence and a great deal of willpower will be needed but, as I've proved myself, it can be done.

When I stopped smoking, some 15 years ago now, it was very, very difficult, I'd been a smoker for over 15 years

---

and I was smoking a pack or more a day, the smokers
who read this will appreciate just how difficult it was, but
once I was over the initial withdrawal problems life
became so much more enjoyable and I had the same
sense of enjoyment, a sense of victory almost, when I
finally learnt to only eat when I was hungry and only to
snack on those foods and drinks which weren't going to
compromise my weight loss goals.

If you will learn to eat only when you're hungry I have
no doubt that with persistence and determination you too
can beat the bad habits and get the body you really want
to have and also get all of the good feelings and health
benefits which go with that.

KEEP A FOOD DIARY.

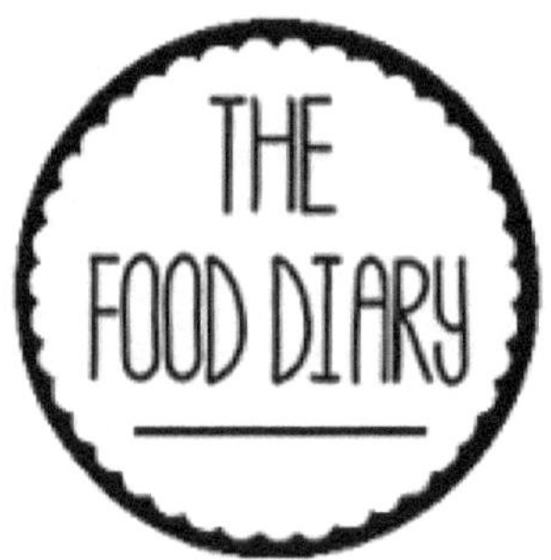

Many people keep a daily diary and each has his or her own reasons for doing so.

As children we're often encouraged to write down things that have happened during our day and to put pen to paper to record our hopes and dreams and our progress towards them.

As we grow and get a job a diary is often a basic requirement, a way of keeping track of appointments, of things we must do and so on.

In fact we're told by those who should know that writing down our goals is the first step to achieving them so it seems to follow that we should be keeping track of our progress when we're losing weight and a food diary is perhaps the best way of doing that.

When you're already keeping a diary for other areas of your life then a food diary is an easy addition to what you're already doing but if, like me, you're not a "diary writer" then it isn't as easy as it sounds.

After all who in their right mind would bother to write down everything they put into their stomach; everything, every day, every minute of every day?

It isn't easy is it?

But just think for a minute, we spend so little time eating that recording what we eat should really take no time at all.

The key here is motivation.

If we have a genuine desire to lose some weight, if we are determined to do so then recording everything we eat and drink shouldn't be a daunting task.

It takes so little time to write down what you had for breakfast, really, how long does it take to write: "2 eggs, 2 rashers of bacon, 1 slice of toast with butter, 2 cups of coffee with sugar".

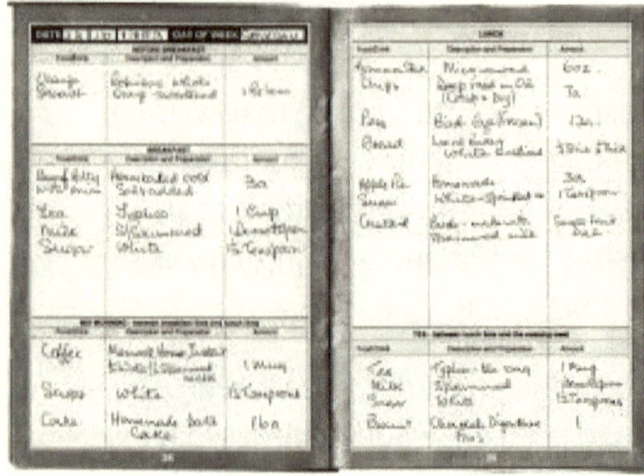

No time at all.

Same for lunch and dinner, such very little time is involved in keeping a food diary that we all should be able to do it without any trouble at all.

If we have the motivation to do so.

So how do get that motivation?

Well perhaps one way could be to have a "fat" picture pasted onto the front cover of our food diary and keep it where it will be seen when we sit down to eat.

If we don't want others to see it put it on the inside of the front cover.

Another way may be to record our weight at the start of each day as the first entry in our food diary for the day, that way we will have a running report on how well our weight loss programme is going.

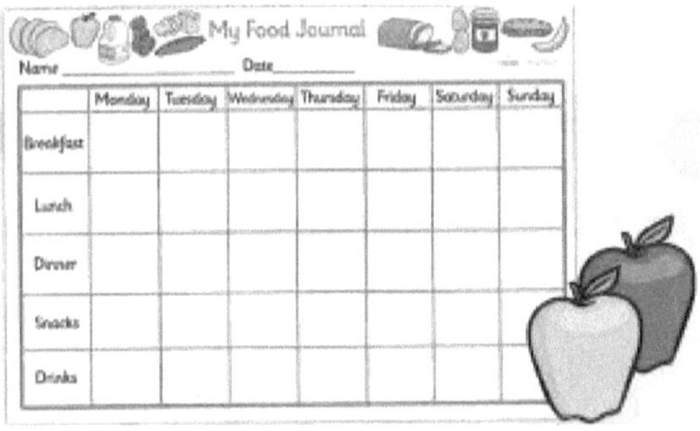

The next thing to determine is what information we should record in our food diary.

The easiest way to do this, at least in the beginning, is to list not only the foods we eat but also the portion sizes.

I don't mean here that we should weight everything as we eat it, that of course isn't practical, but we can give a rough estimate of how much we're eating even if it's only "a large, medium, small" portion.

As we get used to keeping our food diary we might go on to categorise the types of food, is it a vegetable, fruit, red meat, fish and so on.

This information when considered with our recorded weight at the beginning of each day will give us some very good indications as to what is helping us to lose weight and what is hindering us.

It will also be very useful as a tool to help us when we're planning our meals.

Now, we all like to indulge ourselves every so often and there's no need to feel guilty when we do, it helps to keep us on track and prevents us from feeling deprived when we occasionally eat something which we love but which doesn't contribute to our weight loss, the key here is to do so in moderation.

A few bites of that chocolate cake won't derail our efforts, eating the whole cake might do so, but we must make sure we write that down as well, not doing so will be counterproductive and may lead to feelings of guilt.

Another useful "trick" is to reward ourselves when we find that things have gone particularly well, even if it's only a gold star stuck on the page that proves to us that we're doing the right things, it's amazing what extra motivation it will provide as we look back through our food diary to check on our progress.

There is no doubt that for many of us the food diary habit is a challenging one to adopt but once we've made it a daily part of our lives we will find it to be a very worthwhile investment in our weight loss programme.

LEARN TO SAY "NO".

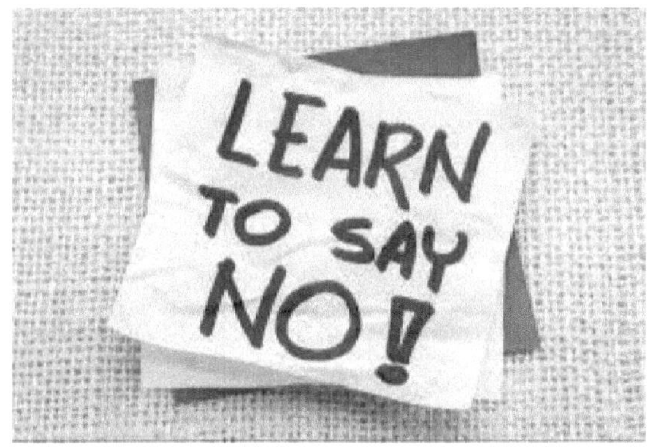

Soon after we were born our parents taught us that it was a really good idea if we didn't say "no".

When we said "yes" we not only got their approval but often we would be rewarded for "being a good girl/boy".

So from the very earliest age saying yes became the accepted way to go.

"Yes" got us the approval of everyone who mattered in our life, in the early days it was our parents then it was our teachers and still later "yes" was what was expected of us by our employer.

Saying "yes" was the way forward; it was really the only way to get ahead.

Saying "yes" became second nature to us, often even when we really wanted to say "no".

It becomes a way of life and I know people who, even in their late 50s and 60s, really hate saying "no" so much that they will agree to almost anything to avoid upsetting someone else.

Now being agreeable is not wrong and in fact it is a really good way to live but only so far as it doesn't negatively impact our own life.

There are definitely times when saying "no" is a much better option and when it comes to food and drink that is certainly the way to go.

If we're out for the evening with family or friends and we're driving for example, it's a really, really good idea to say no to that extra drink, if we don't not only might we lose our licence for driving under the influence but it's not good for our health, the health of those in the car with you and other road users we might come across on our way.

Perhaps we need to start to think in a similar way about our food.

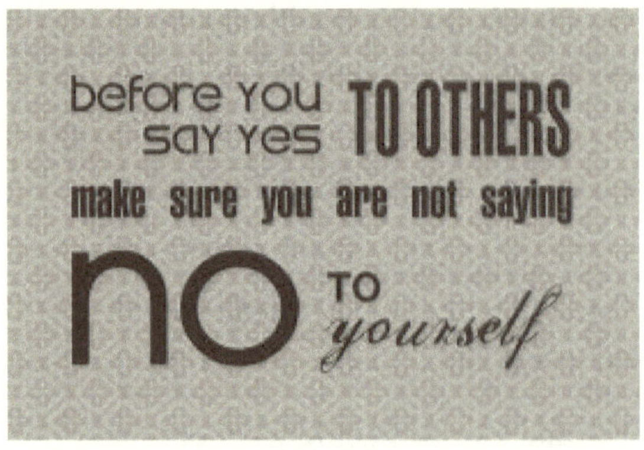

We aren't going to get a ticket for driving having eaten too much at dinner but the consequences could be just as devastating if we do it too often.

Saying "no" however doesn't come easily to most of us, good sales people rely on this fact to help us to purchase all those wonderful things we have in our cupboards but never use.

Saying "no" to an extra helping of dessert when it might offend the maker of that delicious fare isn't easy, it takes some intestinal fortitude and the will to perhaps be a little different to everyone else.

We've probably been taught all of our life that it's easier and more polite to say "yes", to comply with whatever the request is providing it isn't dangerous or illegal, than it is to swim against the tide and say "no" when that's what we really want to say.

But, if we want to control our weight then we must learn to say "no" on the occasions when just agreeing and eating will cause us to stray from our diet just as an alcoholic has to say "no" to that drink when saying "yes" will cause him to fall off the wagon.

Admitting to ourselves that we have a problem saying no is a good place to start, from there we can, with a little practice, become really good at saying no when we want to, it isn't rude it's just us being assertive and telling those around us that we do indeed have a say when it comes to what we want to do, especially when it comes to food.

Learn to say "no", practice it and tell those who would seek to influence our life that we really are the one who's in control, our waistline will thank us for it and our friends and family will quickly learn that when we say "no thank you" we really mean it.

STAYING MOTIVATED.

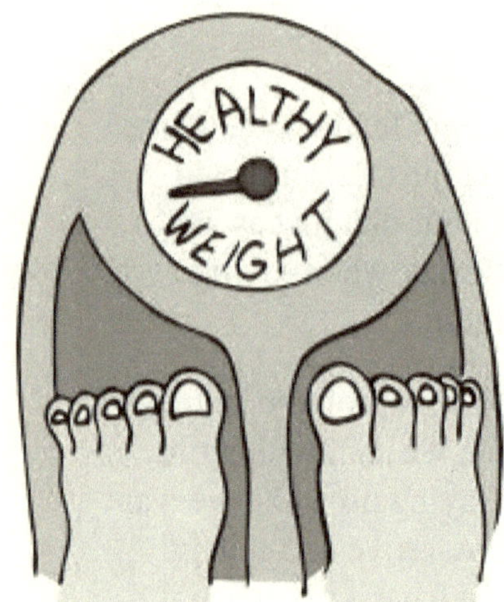

Whenever you are attempting to do something which is new to you or something which is outside your comfort zone staying motivated can be difficult but it is crucial to your success.

No less so when you're attempting to lose weight.

Weight loss motivation however isn't always as easy as looking at that picture of the overweight you which you stuck on the back of the toilet door at the beginning of your journey.

Staying motivated or even getting the motivation to lose weight in the first place, for someone who has spent their adult years avoiding any and all exercise can be very difficult.

Let's face it, if going to the gym or jogging every evening isn't your thing then you won't be able to get excited about it and after a short period you may begin to wonder if all the effort is really worth it.

While starting an exercise programme is easy enough sticking to it isn't so easy and the key here is to determine, right at the start, that, come hell or high water you won't give up.

Perseverance is the key, make a commitment to yourself and determine that you will stick to it just as if you had made a commitment to your significant other, you wouldn't want to let them down so don't let yourself down.

Bear in mind that exercise alone won't get you to your ultimate goal weight but it is a very important part of the process, you don't want to lose 20% of your body weight only to find that what's left is just loose skin and flab!

Having a solid goal helps here and that goal should be something that you can believe you can do, there's no point in setting yourself to lose 5 kilos each week because it's unlikely to happen and you'll get discouraged and probably give up altogether.

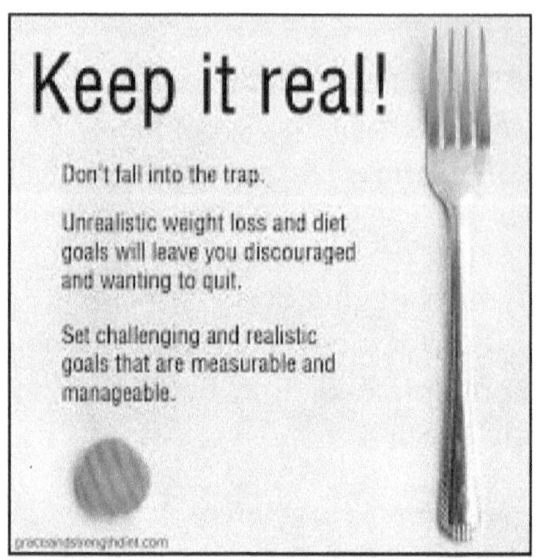

The key to goal setting, whether you're losing weight or doing anything else that requires a goal is to make that goal one which is both believable and, in your mind, achievable.

These short term goals are important but they're only half of the picture you must have a longer term goal as well.

If, for example, your weekly goal is to lose 1 kilo each week your longer term goal might be to lose 20 kilos in the next six months.

Keeping a diary and recording your journey, what you did this week, what you ate, how much exercise you got and, of course, how much weight you lost will provide you with an extra boost of motivation when you're tired and fed up with it all.

You'll be able to read your diary entries and see just how well you're doing, that should give you enough encouragement to get over "the hump".

"The hump" is something, by the way, which everyone who has ever had to work or even struggle to achieve something important has to get over.

It comes generally about a quarter to a third of the way through the journey and presents itself as an almost overwhelming desire to give up and settle for the status quo.

If you have your diary to look back on, to see how far you've come, it provides wonderful encouragement for the next few steps.

You might also consider joining a social group that engages in some form of exercise, you might join a rock and roll dance class, learn belly dancing, play social golf, join the local bush walking group, the opportunities are endless and you're sure to find something you enjoy which will keep you committed.

One last thing on the subject of staying motivated, it is really important to celebrate your successes be they large or small.

Reward yourself for losing that one kilo each week, perhaps, at the end of the month do something special which you really enjoy, buy yourself a new "something" go somewhere special, whatever, but do reward yourself [just don't go to the ice cream parlour and undo all the good work].

Losing weight is a journey and sometimes it's a difficult one, it involves diet and exercise and almost all of the obstacles you'll face on your journey are in your mind, find a way to stay motivated that works for you, don't ever give up, you'll find that as you travel your mind will be transformed into something special and your body will be transformed into something beautiful.

A FEW TIPS TO HELP YOU STAY ON TRACK.

OK, you've made the big decision, you've set your weight loss goals, you've written them down, you've changed the way you eat and you've started to get some decent exercise, now what?

Well what comes next is probably the most difficult part of your whole weight loss program, staying the course.

Here are just a few tips to help you stay on track and win your war against excess weight.

1. First and possibly easiest to do is to remind yourself of the reasons you want to shed the extra kilos.

Write down all the benefits you can think of for losing weight, the benefits to your health, possibly the benefits to your relationships, even the benefits to your bank balance when you don't spend money on things like junk food and sweet treats etc.

If you have one put a photo of the "big" you somewhere you can see it often, if you don't want anyone else to see it stick it in your closet or on the back of your toilet door and next to it put the written list of your reasons for losing weight. Look at them often, you'll be amazed how much motivation you'll get from looking at them several times each day.

2. Get hold of some small cards, business card size would be good, and write on them some positive affirmations, words or phrases that will remind you why you're losing weight.

Write your affirmations as though you have already achieved your goal weight, for example you might write "I feel so much healthier now that I weigh only [xx] kilos", avoid phrases that still put you at your current weight or that suggest that you're "trying" to lose weight.

Why small cards?

Well you can carry them in your pocket or bag and no-one else has to see them but you' be able to refer to them any time you wish.

Another important thing about affirmations, they won't work if you just read them to yourself, you must voice them so that you can hear them yourself, with your ears!

3. Practice seeing yourself slim.

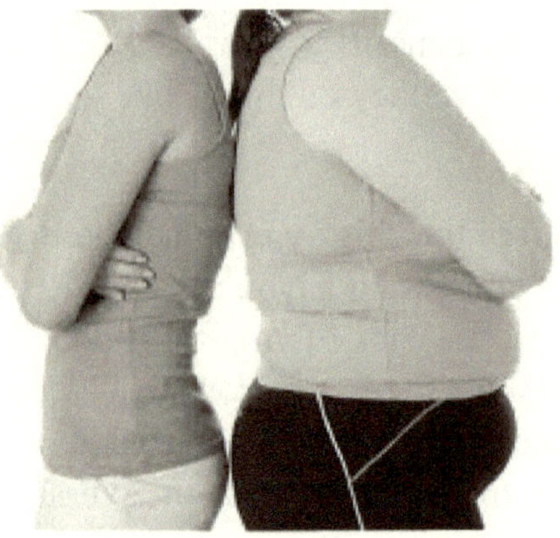

Silly as it might sound seeing yourself how you really want to be, visualisation is the "proper" term, will make it easier for you to reach your goal weight.

Visualise how you will feel when you are your goal weight, imagine what your friends and family will say, see yourself enjoying all the things you will have when you're slim.

But for this to be a part of your success you need to actually "feel" it, it's not going to help if you just think about it, you really need to feel it for visualisation to be of any help.

4. Decide for yourself what habits you will need to adopt in order to lose weight.

Will it help if you only cook good wholesome food and forget your deep fryer?

What about getting into a regular exercise routine or taking a different route to work to avoid the patisserie that bakes those delicious Danish pastries?

If you think about it you will know what habits you need to ditch and which ones you should adopt.

It may be hard to change what you've been doing [and enjoying] for years but in order for you to attain your goal weight you are going to have to do something other than what you have been doing, after all, what you have been doing has got you where you are today.

If you change what you do and continue with the change for 30 days you will have formed a new habit, a much better one.

If you make a mistake and go back into the old habits then your 30 days will have to start again, it's hard I know but the results are well worth the effort.

5. Organise your time a little better so that you have more time for exercise and for cooking good food.

Take-away food generally is not the healthiest, most fast food is cooked in too much fat and sits around in a hot box until someone buys it and I know exercise takes time but you don't have to watch DOOL on the box every day and you don't really need 5 news fixes every day do you?

Take time off from the TV and go to the gym, leave the car in the garage and walk to the local shop, play outside with your children, they'll make you run and you'll be better for it.

Finally fight any temptation to give up on your desire to lose weight.

You may have some bad days along the way, days when you eat one Tim Tam too many, when you just can't sum up the energy to go for your evening walk but we all have days when things just don't work out as we planned.

Don't give up, remember the old saying "when the going gets tough the tough get going", pull out your little cards with your affirmations written on them, remember the reasons for wanting to lose weight in the first place, look at that picture of the "big" you and ask yourself what you want more, to go back to being over-weight and un-healthy or to build yourself that new, slim, svelte body that you've wanted for so long.

Don't give up, keep working at it, you can do it.

WEIGHT LOSS TIPS THAT ACTUALLY WORK.

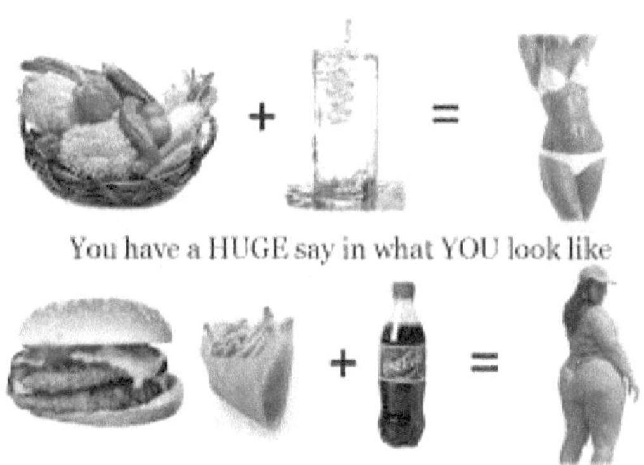

It doesn't seem to matter where you look these days there's a new weight loss tip or weight loss program that's "guaranteed" to help you lose weight fast.

Every women's magazine has at least one weight loss tip, every chemist shop has row upon row of weight loss pills and supplements, every gym we go to is promoting this or that weight loss product but does anybody know what actually works for weight loss?

It seems the answer to that question is a definite "yes".

The boffins who study obesity and its fixes have declared that there are six weight loss tips that actually work and these six weight loss tips will, if we take notice of them, give us a better than average chance of losing weight, regaining control of our appetite and getting the body we deserve.

So what are these six weight loss tips?

Read on!

1. The first thing we need to realise is that we can't lose too much weight by just exercising but we must also change our diet.

In fact, according to Dr. Samuel Klein MD, at Washington University's School of Medicine, limiting our calorie intake is a much more effective way to lose weight than exercising.

Taking the stairs instead if the lift is a good idea for our general health and fitness but it won't do much for our waist line.

If we run 5 kilometres [3 miles] we'll probably burn something like 300 calories, a lot of effort for so little reward when we can just not eat one bag of potato chips and get the same result.

The exercise may also have the negative effect, as far as weight loss is concerned, of increasing our appetite.

When we exercise we stimulate our hunger hormones and, let's face it, there's not much point in running or working out for an hour if we then go home and eat a pizza washed down with a glass of beer.

There are other factors involved here as well, when we exercise our bodies compensate, they're very good at that, we get tired and are more likely to do less for the rest of the day thereby negating the effects of the exercise.

So, diet beats exercise for weight loss but both together really do the job so much better.

2. Food combinations have little effect when it comes to weight loss.

We've been told that when we discover the right combination of foods for our body type it will, as if by magic, help us to shed the kilos.

It won't!

There is no magic formula when it comes to the food we eat, regardless of the type of diet we employ it's always going to be the calories that make it a success or failure.

There is no evidence to suggest that any particular diet will work better with a particular body type or metabolic make-up.

It's a myth, perpetrated by those who have something to gain, that there is some specific combination of foods which will suit our individual metabolism.

Science has proven that almost any decent diet will work for almost everybody as long as we follow it!

3. Regardless of how we get it a calorie is still a calorie.

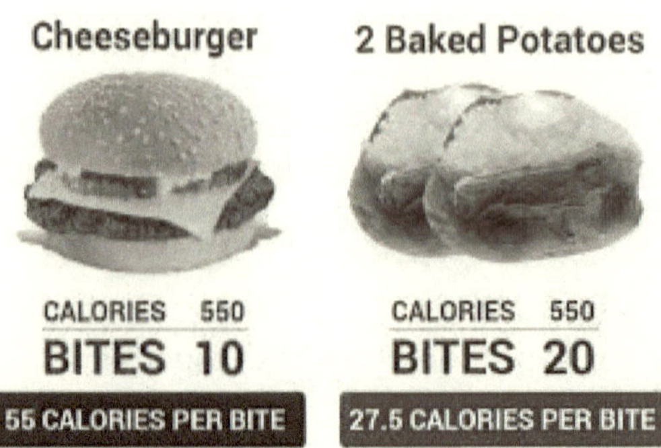

Most of us have read about the "junk food diet" which was undertaken by Professor Mark Haub at Kansas State University.

During a ten week period the professor, who has a Masters in Exercise Science and a PhD in Exercise Physiology, apparently lost about 10 kilos over a period of 10 weeks by just eating "junk food".

Sounds impressive, and it is but, and it's a big but [pardon the pun] while the professor was on his "junk food diet" he still limited his calorie intake to about 33% less calories than his normal diet or a diet considered normal for a man of his weight and height.

It also was supplemented with some healthy, nutritional foods such as celery sticks and green beans and he took a multi-vitamin and a nutritional shake each day.

The point here is that if we were to be silly enough to read the part of the story which says that a well credentialed university professor lost 10 kilos by just eating junk food we'd be doing ourselves no good at all.

Obviously it wasn't the junk food that caused the weight loss it was the fact that at about 97 kilos he was grossly over-weight to start with and he severely limited his calorie intake.

Junk food is not good for us, it has some very nasty addictions associated with it but even just eating junk food, if we limit the calories involved we will lose weight.

As I said above, a calorie is a calorie is a calorie.

4. A broken metabolism???

Is that even possible???

It seems that the answer is "yes".

For years doctors have told us that a broken metabolism is not a medical possibility, it now appears that they were wrong and we can indeed have a metabolism which doesn't work as it should.

Scientists have discovered, from research out of NASA, that periods of inactivity such as experienced by astronauts causes our metabolism to slow down and become inflexible, in effect it becomes "broken".

How can we fix this?

If we start to become active our metabolism does improve so physical exercise is the answer, if we've been inactive for a long period of time we may never get our metabolism back to working as it should but we will go a long way towards it.

Apart from the other reasons for exercising, after we've lost some of that excess weight exercise will help us to maintain the weight loss by boosting our metabolism, that's another good reason to get active.

5. To follow on from the point above, if we've been sedentary for a long time the it is entirely possible that our metabolism may never return to its former state before we became overweight and inactive.

The uncomfortable take-away from this is that even though we begin to exercise again and our metabolism begins to return we may never be in a position where we can slack off a bit.

If our metabolism has slowed to any great degree we will probably have to work harder for longer to see and maintain any weight loss benefits.

It isn't a nice reality but it is something we must come to terms with in order to not get frustrated when we see others not doing it so tough and still getting the results.

Unfair as it may seem it's just something we have to accept and learn to live with.

6. Finally for this post, our brains are the over-riding influencers when it comes to us being overweight or slim.

Certainly our metabolism plays a part but our bodies only reflect what we decide, with our brains, to do to them.

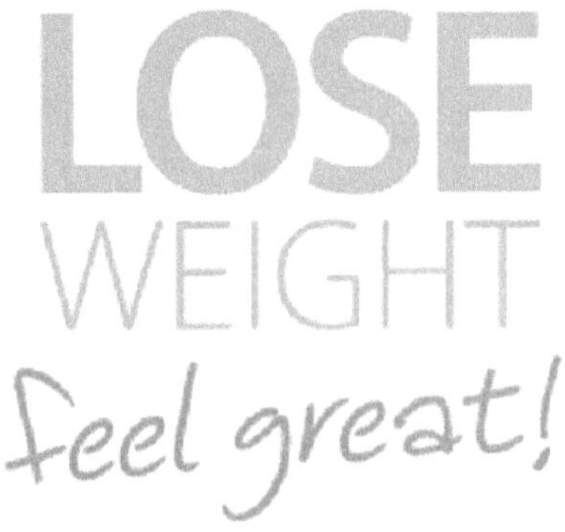

Poor decisions regarding food and exercise are the primary causes of obesity unless, of course, we have a physical or hormonal condition which we can't control and over a period of time, in my case a period of many years, we teach our brains to behave in a certain way and it then becomes "normal" to eat this way, to do this or that thing, the patterns are established and so become very difficult to change.

The good news here is that the brain can be re-programmed, when we embark upon a changed lifestyle, over a period of about three weeks or so our brains will start to interpret that changed lifestyle as the new norm making it easier to maintain.

Starting a new diet or exercise program is never easy but it becomes more so the more we stick at it, it make take some time to establish the new patterns of behaviour but it can be done, all it takes is the desire to do so.

If we stick with it we have nothing to lose except our excess weight.

WHEN FAST WEIGHT LOSS BECOMES UNHEALTHY.

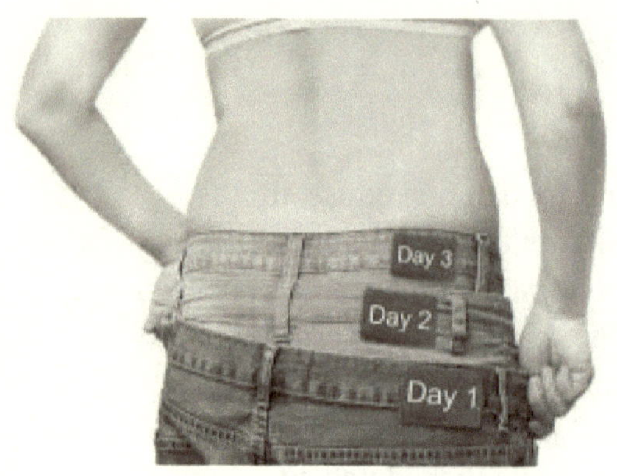

So you've made the decision to lose weight as quickly as possible, you have your diet in place and you expect to follow it conscientiously.

At this point, you may be wondering how much weight you can lose in a given week and whether fast weight loss can be detrimental for your body.

There are however a number of things that can affect your weight loss.

Family history and genetics can play a significant role, your fast weight loss will probably depend, to a significant degree, upon how much exercise you're engaging in as well as how much stress you are under and your metabolism, or how quickly you burn calories, will also have a major effect.

Theoretically, you could lose as much as 5 to 8 kilos a week however much of that weight could be water weight.

So what is "water weight" and why is it important?

Well according to the experts, "water weight", simply put, is the weight that results from your body retaining excess water.

An estimated 50 to 60 percent of our total body weight is water, and how much we retain changes in response to our eating habits.

If, like me, you enjoy in salty foods or use a lot of salt in your cooking, it can cause your body to hold onto water like a sponge.

In the same way, a diet high in sugar can lead to higher-than-normal insulin levels in your blood, which again can make your body retain sodium [salt] and therefore water.

Do you love pasta?

Well don't we all, but for every gram of carbohydrate [from that pasta for example] your body stores it also stores up three grams of water.

What this means for you is that once you go off your diet, you will probably gain much of that weight back.

Also, unless you engage in some form of muscle building exercise you will be losing muscle as well as fat since about a quarter of your body's weight consists of muscle.

It is interesting to note that, again according to the experts, the most you can safely lose is about two kilos of fat in any given week.

Your body has a way of protecting itself against extreme weight loss, so if your calorie count suddenly drops, your body will compensate by reducing your metabolic rate.

As a result you'll need fewer calories to maintain your weight.

Gets confusing doesn't it?

This explains why you may lose weight up to a point and then be unable to lose any extra weight, no matter how hard you try.

Blame Mother Nature!

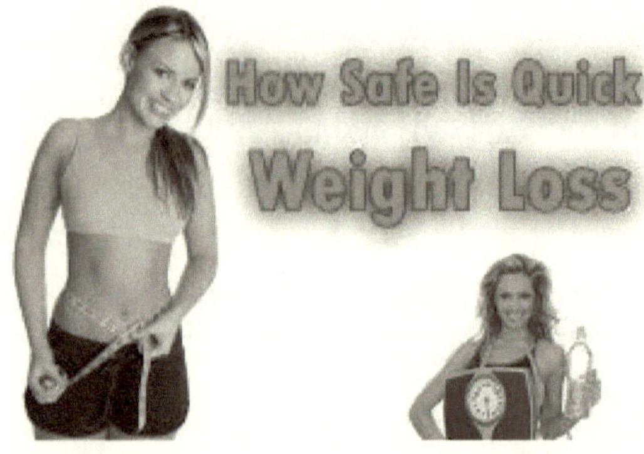

Also if you lose weight quickly, there's a good chance that your health may be compromised.

Fast weight loss has been linked to the formation of gall stones, you may experience loose skin as your weight goes into free fall and perhaps most distressing of all, if you experience fast weight loss, there's a good chance that you will gain the weight back again.

Fast weight loss also places you at greater risk for an eating disorder, you may be tempted to starve yourself, leading to anorexia or, because your food cravings are so great, you may want to binge and purge, leading to a case of bulimia.

This is why for many people it is so vitally important to lose weight under the care of a physician otherwise you could be doing more harm to your body than good.

Although the body has the capability of shedding a great deal of weight over a period of time, most medical experts agree that one should not expect to lose more than a kilo or two a week in order to remain healthy.

This can be disappointing to a dieter, especially one that needs to lose a significant amount of weight, however, doctors believe that the go-slow approach is best for long-term weight loss otherwise you could end up with a number of health problems you weren't expecting.

On the positive side there are a number of approaches you can use to lose weight.

You might follow one of any number of diets which are freely available on the internet, diets like the Atkins plan, the Zone, or the diabetic diet, you might try Sugar Busters or the Carb Addict's prescription for losing weight but however you decide to lose your weight it is vitally important that you accompany your diet plan with an effective exercise routine.

One of the best exercises you can do, in fact, is the easiest, and that is walking.

It has been said that you can lose as much as a kilo a week, just by walking alone.

As we have explained here fast weight loss should be undertaken with caution.

It is far better to shed a kilo or two each week and maintain that weight loss over the long term.

All good things take time, and that is particularly true when it comes to weight loss so perhaps the best advice is to be patient, follow a reasonable diet, get plenty of exercise, and drink a good amount of water.

That way, you should be able to slowly lose weight— without jeopardizing your health in the process.

WHY BREAKFAST IS SO IMPORTANT.

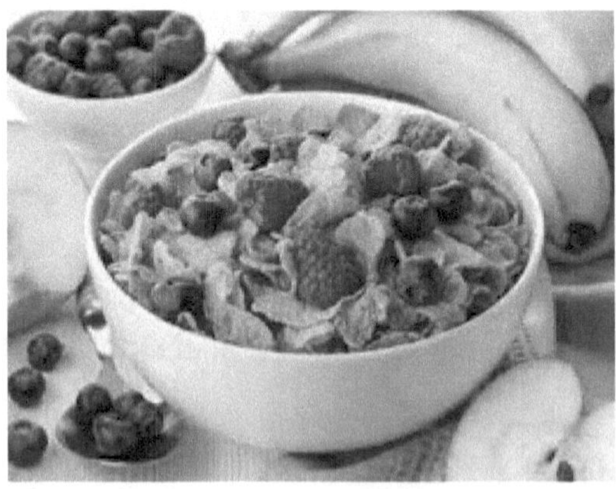

Many of us wake in the morning, head straight for that early fix with a cup or two of coffee, shower, get dressed for the day and then realise that we don't have time to sit and eat breakfast.

We might grab a slice or two of toast and tell ourselves that's all we need, after all we're on a diet aren't we and the less we eat the better.

Wrong!

If this is you then you're doing yourself much more harm than good.

There are a number of very good reasons to eat breakfast, particularly if you are a dieter.

For a start, eating at the start of your day, regardless of what time that is, will speed up your metabolism and that is a critical factor in your effort to lose weight.

When you think about it, you generally eat dinner sometime early evening and if you wait to eat again until lunch the next day that's often about 18 hours between food intakes.

That's not good for you.

Also, by missing out on breakfast you may have a tendency to eat a bigger lunch than you should which doesn't help in your efforts to lose weight.

There are any number of scientific studies to show that those who eat breakfast are in the great majority when it comes to losing weight.

It seems to go against logical thinking that in order to lose weight you should eat more food but that "logic" definitely does not apply when it comes to breakfast.

As an aside, and while it has little to do with losing weight, eating breakfast has been shown to aid concentration and improve your ability to focus which is a definite advantage for those who are studying or who have jobs that require a great deal of mental agility.

Having said all of the above, breakfast is not just something to put into your stomach at the start of the day.

The type of food you eat is also very important.

Your breakfast should preferably be primarily a high fibre meal or a meal which is full of protein and should contain plenty of vitamins and minerals to help you remain healthy right through the day.

Avoid sugary sweet things like most packaged breakfast cereals which many of us tend to add more sugar to anyway.

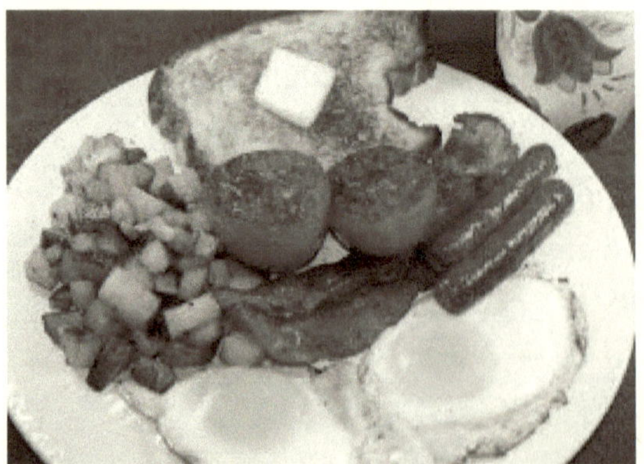

That type of breakfast will give you a short lift in your energy levels due to the sugar but will do you no good in the long run.

Another good reason to eat a healthy breakfast is that will lift your mood, something that is very important when it comes to dieting and losing weight.

It's easy to get down when you're dieting and anything which will help to overcome that without jeopardising your weight loss goal has to be a good thing.

Breakfast is the first meal decision of your day, if you make good choices at breakfast then you are much more likely to make good meal decisions for the rest of the day and while it is better to eat something rather that nothing you should be careful in the food choices you make at breakfast.

One thing that must be avoided is treating breakfast as an opportunity to over-indulge.

The thinking might be that if you eat a good breakfast you could skip other meals during the day and this is not a good idea.

For your body to be at its best it needs regular intakes of nourishment, healthy meals at reasonably regular intervals and depending on whose advice you follow this may mean three meals a day or it may mean five or six smaller meals.

Last but by no means least you must realise that eating breakfast is a habit and like any other habit, good or bad, it takes some time to get into it.

Persistence is the key here, eat something for breakfast *every* morning, if need be start with a small helping of something healthy, make sure you actually sit down and eat, don't take breakfast on the run, if necessary write it into your schedule for the day and make sure you do it.

Start a good habit and after about a month it will be so ingrained into your thinking that you'll just do it.

THE SECRETS TO WEIGHT LOSS AFTER PREGNANCY.

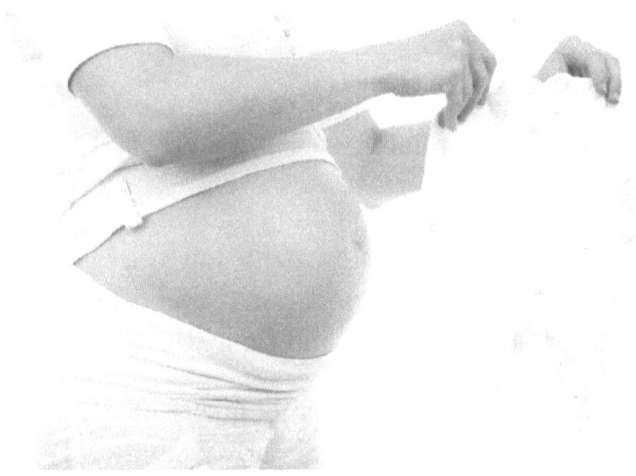

So, you've just had your third baby and you're concerned that you may not be able to lose your baby weight.

After both of your previous pregnancies you have had difficulty losing your baby weight and with all of your other responsibilities weight loss isn't a major concern at the moment however once your baby is born, like most other women you would very much like to return to your pre-pregnancy weight.

The average woman gains more than 10 kilos during her pregnancy and although the very act of giving birth may result in a weight loss of up to 5 – 6 kilos, new moms still have considerable weight to lose once they leave the hospital.

Some women take the easy option and simply assume that this "baby fat" is now a permanent part of their life and they will never get rid of it but it is entirely possible to lose some, or all, of this baby weight during the after birth period.

Most doctors will recommend easing into a weight loss program after the birth of your baby.

This means that you should not start dieting until about three months after the birth of your new baby and you should combine a low-fat diet with moderate exercise in order to regain your pre-birth weight [and figure].

Don't expect instant results, it will probably take you a good nine months to get back to your pre baby weight.

After childbirth your body needs time to recover so it's a good idea to take it slowly in your efforts to lose weight.

You could almost certainly lose weight faster but you might be sacrificing valuable nutrients as a result.

There is also some reliable evidence to indicate that breastfeeding actually helps with weight loss.

The American College of Obstetricians and Gynaecologists has found that breastfeeding leads to the release of hormones which allow your uterus to return to its normal size.

Breastfeeding alone however won't bring down your weight; you will need to combine it with a sensible diet and a reasonable exercise program [without overdoing it].

Remember that you need to have a minimum of 1800 calories a day whilst breastfeeding in order to keep yourself and your baby healthy.

You should really only eat food with high nutritional value to maintain the proper level of calories each day.

There are a host of good reasons to exercise at any time but it is equally important during the period immediately after the birth.

In addition to helping to accelerate weight reduction, exercise can help alleviate "after birth blues", improve your mood and boost your confidence.

Exercise can also help you to think more clearly so that you're better able to meet the demands of motherhood.

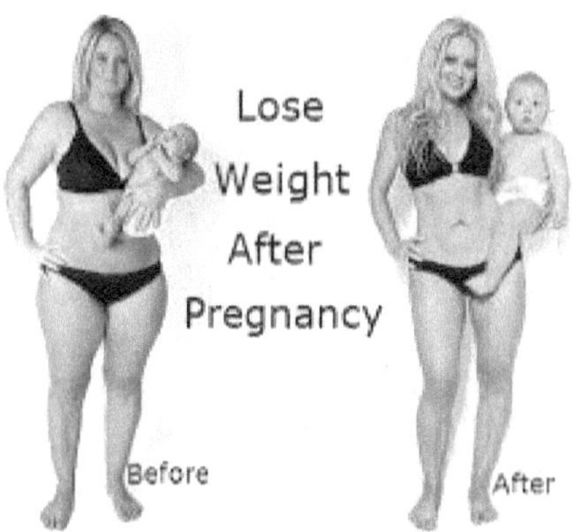

You might consider joining an exercise class that caters for new mothers so that your baby can cxcrcisc right along with you or you might enlist the help of a friend or relative to exercise with you so that you'll have some emotional support while exercising.

An added benefit of working out is that it should increase your energy levels which is quite important when battling the weariness which comes from caring for a newborn.

Your diet should generally be low-fat but not fat-free; vitamin rich and high in fibre.

Under no circumstances should you go on a fad diet.

Fad diets are never a good idea, could be quite harmful to your health and could actually slow your recovery from childbirth.

Also it's a good idea to set achievable weight-loss goals, with the emphasis on "achievable".

Recognize that there's a limit to the amount of weight you can lose during a given period of time especially after your pregnancy.

You will undoubtedly see a number of celebrity moms on the covers of magazines shortly after the birth of their children, they appear slender and elegant, totally devoid of baby fat [hey, you can look like that too, just photo shop your pics like they do].

In the accompanying article they may even talk about exercising right after childbirth.

These articles send new mothers a dangerous message, that you should do all you can to become thin as quickly as possible after your baby is born.

Such a viewpoint is not only ridiculous it's also bad for you.

Therefore you'll need to ignore those messages from the media, treat them for what they are and stay the course with your own gradual weight loss plan.

The time right after the birth of your baby can be quite challenging, taxing both your physical and emotional strength.

You do need to eat healthy, for both yourself and your new baby, but it's important to pace yourself as far as weight loss is concerned.

Over time, you will be able to lose the baby weight you gained during your pregnancy and you might find that you're actually healthier after your baby is born than you were before.

Just be sensible and lose your baby weight in a healthy way.

WEIGHT LOSS - MYTHS AND MISCONCEPTIONS.

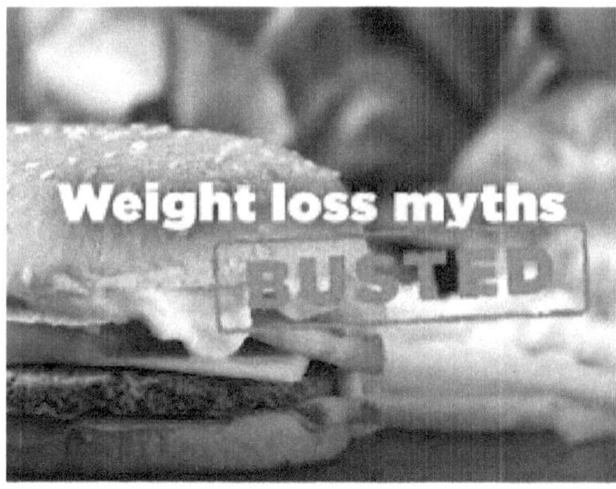

When it comes to weight loss many of us are prepared to believe almost anything which [according to the advertising] offers us an easy and pain free solution to being overweight.

This can be a very dangerous situation because much of that which is touted as being the miracle solution to our weight problems can actually be quite detrimental to our health.

Obviously the better informed we are regarding the myths that abound in the weight loss industry the better we will be to make the good decisions which need to be made.

So, what are some of these myths?

Well, one of the most misleading is that anything which is labelled as "natural" must be safe, however nature abounds with things which are not safe for human consumption and often these "natural" products undergo no scientific testing whatsoever.

As an example, Ephedra and products like it have been linked to serious health problems and even death.

To borrow from The Mayo Clinic's website:

http://www.mayoclinic.org/drugs-supplements/ephedra--ma-huang/background/hrb-20059270

"In 2003, there was a death of a U.S. major league baseball pitcher which was thought to be related to Ephedra. The U.S. Food and Drug Administration (FDA) has collected more than 800 reports of serious toxicity, including more than 22 deaths. On February 6, 2004, the FDA issued a rule prohibiting the sale of dietary supplements containing ephedrine alkaloids (Ephedra).

This rule was issued because supplements with Ephedra present a serious risk of illness or injury.

In 2005 this rule was struck down in Utah but reversed again four months later. Ephedra is currently banned throughout the United States. It remains unclear whether Ephedra will re-appear on the market, despite serious safety risks, including heart events or death."

Ephedra is currently banned in the USA yet we still find it in some weight loss supplements, makes you wonder....

Consulting with our medical professional before we take ANY weight loss supplements is a really good idea.

Another myth we need to be careful about is that if a product is labelled as "low fat" or "fat free" it won't cause us a problem with our weight.

Many such products have just as many calories in them as the standard variety and they also often contain high proportions of sugar and flour which increase the calorie count.

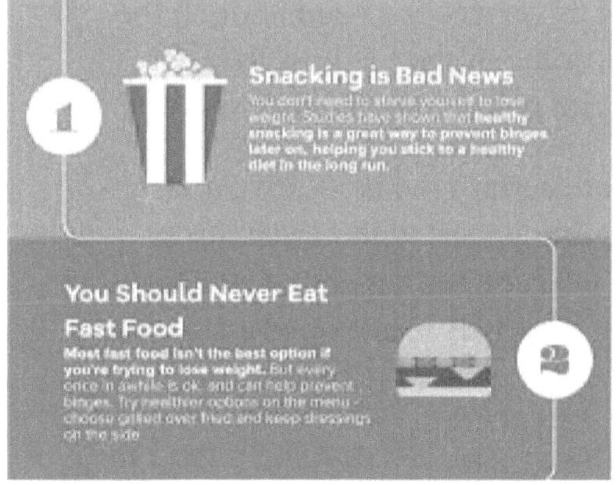

It's important that we read the nutritional label on the food we buy to determine the exact amount of calories in a standard serving and also to determine what constitutes a "standard" serve.

Another common myth is that we can eat as we please and still lose weight by increasing our exercise.

We see all the time overweight people in the gym or jogging along the street believing that just an increase in physical activity will somehow magically cause them to lose those extra kilos.

It won't!

Without some control of the food we consume we are destined to an ongoing struggle with our weight.

Yes exercise is an important part of our weight loss programme but exercise alone won't give us the long term weight loss results we're all looking for.

We need to change the way we eat, we need to ditch the old habits, possibly with some of the food we have grown to love and cultivate new eating habits.

We all know that there are certain foods we love and other foods we don't like but just as with our children when they were young, we kept putting greens on their plate at dinner until they eventually developed a taste for them.

We too, in our more mature years, can develop a taste for almost anything if we stick with it for long enough.

Perhaps the old adage that says "there's no gain without pain" is appropriate here; we should endure the "pain" of eating what we don't like until we come to like it, to get the "gain" of achieving our weight loss goals.

Now how about fast foods.

Is it possible to eat at MacDonalds and still lose weight?

Yes, of course it is!

The trick is to be careful what you order, to pay attention to your portion size [perhaps sharing the fries etc. with a friend] obviously don't order the super size combo and drink water instead of coke.

Many fast food outlets today also offer a less fattening alternative, a chicken sandwich instead of a whopper, a Caesar salad rather than a hot dog with the lot and leave the mayo and melted cheese alone, your meal will be just as enjoyable as, and far less fattening than, the traditional fast food fare.

There are so many myths and misconceptions about food that I could write a book about it, [perhaps I will one day], here I've mentioned just a few, the important thing is to be sensible and if in doubt consult your doctor or dietician before embarking on any weight loss regime.

WHAT THE UNITED STATES GOVERNMENT SAYS ABOUT WEIGHT LOSS.

You may well be surprised that the US government has any opinion at all on the subject of weight loss let alone actually *what* it has to say!

The US National Institute of Health which is, of course, part of the US government has some very interesting ideas on what it takes to slim down and shed the kilos.

You may also be surprised to learn that these ideas often disagree with what you'll read in the popular press.

If you've been dieting or trying to lose weight for any time at all you will no doubt have heard that you should avoid, or at least limit your intake of red meat.

You will have read that eating red meat makes it more difficult to lose the weight however lean red meat can actually be a critical component of a healthy diet.

While red meat, together with chicken and pork may have saturated fats and cholesterol they also contain important minerals which are needed for your body to operate as it should.

It is important however that the meat you consume is low in fat, round steak, sirloin and flank are good, and you should also be conscious of your portion size, which will, of course, depend on your build, a smaller person will need a smaller portion.

You will have heard that most dairy products are fattening but the low fat varieties have all the nutrients of the regular products without the calories and most of the fat.

Dairy products provide you with a good deal of calcium, protein and vitamin D all of which are essential for good health.

Economic Cost of Obesity

PREVALENCE OF OVERWEIGHT AND OBESITY IN AMERICA

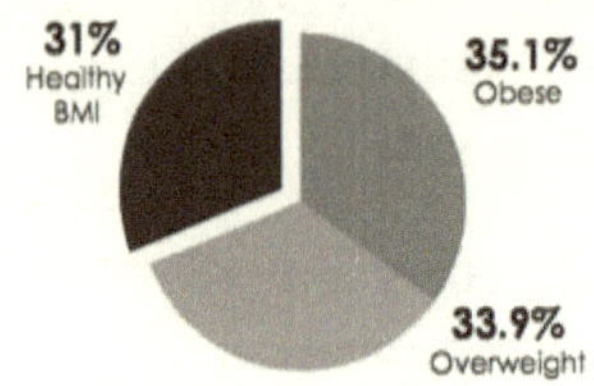

2 in 3 adults are overweight or obese. 1

OBESITY CAUSES

Heart disease and stroke
High blood pressure
High Cholesterol
Diabetes
Some cancers

$ The cost to your bottom line

$190.2 BILLION — The estimated annual health care costs of obesity-related illness.[2]

$4.3 BILLION — The cost of obesity-related job absenteeism annually.[3]

$506 PER YEAR PER OBESE WORKER — Obesity is associated with lower productivity (presenteeism) while at work, which costs employers $506 per obese worker per year.[3]

36% HIGHER — Medical costs attributed to obese and overweight adults are 36% higher than those of normal weight.[4]

As a person's BMI increases, so do the number of sick days, medical claims and healthcare costs associated with that person.[3]

WE MAKE HEALTH REWARDING for you and your employees

The average incentaHEALTH participant after one year in the program sees a weight improvement of **5.7%** or **11.7 lbs**

A 5-7% weight loss can prevent the onset of type 2 diabetes

*incenta*HEALTH ™

For more information visit **www.incentaHEALTH.com**

1 www.niddk.nih.gov   2 www.healthycommunitieshealthyfuture.org   3 www.stateofobesity.org   4 www.livewellcolorado.org

According to the US federal guidelines children, teenagers and older people should have at least three servings of dairy per day and those in between, say aged between 20 and 50 years, should have two servings per day, where a "serving" consists of one cup of milk or yoghurt or between 25 and 50 grams of cheese.

If dairy products upset your system you could try the lactose free varieties and you can get your calcium from juice or fish and your vitamin D direct from the sunlight just don't get too much sun, which in itself is not healthy.

You might have considered becoming a vegetarian in the belief that not eating meat will help you to lose weight, the fed however, says that becoming a vegetarian will not automatically help you to shed the kilos.

Studies have indicated that vegetarians do consume less calories that those who eat meat and they tend to have a lower body mass index but even vegetarians have to watch their consumption of high calorie foods.

Another possible problem with a vegetarian diet is a lack of essential minerals and vitamins such as iron, calcium, protein and vitamin D which can be missing from such an eating regime.

It is therefore essential for the vegetarian to find other ways to get what they need, selecting foods which are not only low in fat but also high in nutrition is crucial.

A way to do this is to choose things like green vegetables such as broccoli and spinach for your iron and calcium, eggs are good for vitamin B12 and protein and whole grains offer a whole heap of benefits.

Nuts, no not you ☺, are probably on your hit list, they contain high levels of fat, however a small quantity of nuts can help with your weight loss plan as the fat they contain is not the kind that will clog up your arteries, it is actually healthy fat!

Nuts will provide you with protein, fibre and magnesium but don't overdo it, about one quarter to one half a cup a day is sufficient.

The government health department is adamant that fasting is one of the least effective ways to lose weight, regular but smaller meals, possibly eaten more often, is a much more successful, and healthier, way to go.

Food helps to get your metabolism moving and keeps it going throughout the day.

Does the US government, or any government for that matter, have all the answers for weight loss?

Of course not but it obvious that governments all around the developed world have an acute interest in the health of their citizens and as such all have research departments continually investigating the various claims made by those promoting weight loss programmes as well as providing their own nutritional information.

As these government bodies generally have no commercial interest in weight loss programmes it is reasonable to assume that the information you get from such government sources is information you can trust and taking notice of it could well be beneficial as far as your own weight loss programme is concerned.

If you are unsure about a particular weight loss claim, you can check the US Federal Trade Commission's website at www.ftc.gov/bcp/conline/features/wgtloss.htm for the information you need.

PART TWO – DIETS.

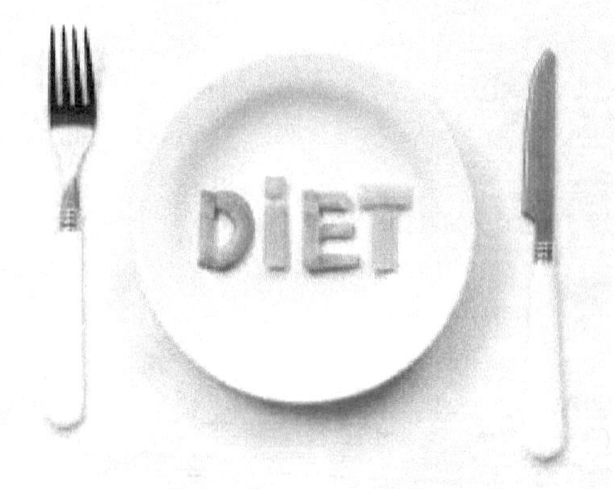

We all know there are diets and there are diets, as with most other things in life not all diets are created equal.

Every year we hear of a new "super weight loss diet" that's "guaranteed" to make you lose those unwanted kilos in the blink of an eye and with no effort on your part.

Many of us have been sucked into buying this and trying that, desperate in the hope that this one will be the diet plan that will see us finally reach those weight loss goals that we so desperately need in our lives.

There are however some very good, well researched and scientifically proven weight loss diets that actually work for many people and these are definitely worth our consideration when we're trying to lose weight.

There are also several different types of diet that we should consider when we're looking to lose weight and understanding each of these would probably be a good place to start on the road to a slimmer body and better health.

Here are just a few of the more accepted diets which have proven to be successful for many others over the years, perhaps one of these is your answer.

THE ATKINS METHOD/DIET.

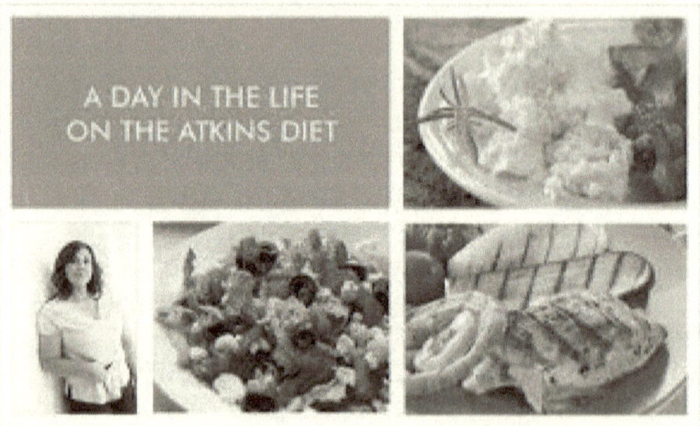

Over the years, the Atkins plan has become synonymous with weight loss. Fans of the program say that it has proven to be instrumental in helping them to shed unwanted pounds. They talk of improved overall health and greater energy as a result of the Atkins program.

However, critics maintain that Atkins could lead to heart damage, making it an unhealthy diet.

Supporters of Atkins say just about anyone can slim down using their program. However, there are certain people that are most likely to benefit from the Atkins plan. These include yo-yo dieters, who find themselves losing weight, only to gain it back again; dieters who feel constantly hungry; and those who eat for emotional reasons.

Binge eaters and constant snackers can also benefit from the Atkins program. In addition, those who suffer from a food addiction are prime candidates for Atkins.

Atkins relies heavily on proteins and fats, along with carbohydrates that are rich in nutrients. The idea is to strictly reduce the amount of non-nutritious carbohydrates you consume. The theory behind this is that, when carbs are restricted, you end up burning fat rather than glucose. In addition, it has been shown that, all things being equal, you will lose more fat with Atkins than with other types of weight loss plans.

The Atkins plan is divided into four stages. During the initial stage, your body moves from burning carbohydrates to burning fats. You should also be able to kick the sugar habit during this stage. During the second stage, your weight loss will accelerate, but you will also be able to eat larger portions of vegetables. In the third stage, known as pre-maintenance, you will continue to add more foods to the mix.

The final stage involves lifetime maintenance. During this phase, you can continue to fight food addictions, maintain your goal weight, and decrease the chance that you will suffer from diabetes.

However, it can be difficult to stick with the Atkins plan. This is because the temptation to eat carbohydrates and sweets is so great. Friends and relatives can become diet saboteurs, preventing you from achieving the results you're looking for. In this case, the best defence is a good offence. This means telling your significant others in advance that you're determined to complete the Atkins program. Inform them that you don't want to even be offered French fries and potato chips.

The Journal of the American Medical Association has suggested that the Atkins plan can be dangerous for children. This is not surprising, considering that young people are still growing and need all the nutrients they can get, whether the vitamins and minerals are from carbohydrates or other sources.

Supporters of Atkins say that, while children may not benefit from a restriction of vegetables and fruits, they could consume fewer potatoes and breads and still remain healthy.

Some medical experts say that the Atkins approach is not appropriate for people who already suffer from kidney or liver trouble. Also, because Atkins reduces the amount of fruits and vegetables an individual consumes, the diet can leave people at greater risk for such problems as cancer and heart disease. As a result, you should probably check with your family physician before resorting to the Atkins plan, or any other low-carb, high-protein diet.

It is likely that the Atkins plan will remain controversial for the foreseeable future. While it has been proven effective in helping people lose weight, it may also place individuals at a higher risk for serious diseases. A great deal of additional research needs to be conducted in order to determine if Atkins is a miracle cure or a medical nightmare.

Once more studies are conducted, the long-term effects of Atkins on the human body may be easier to determine. If you are generally in good health and have a normal energy level, you might give Atkins a try. If, however, you suffer from any serious diseases, or are experiencing symptoms such as high blood pressure, you might consider an alternative diet plan. In the end, you, in consultation with your doctor, will have to determine the diet program that's appropriate in your particular case.

THE LOW CALORIE DIET.

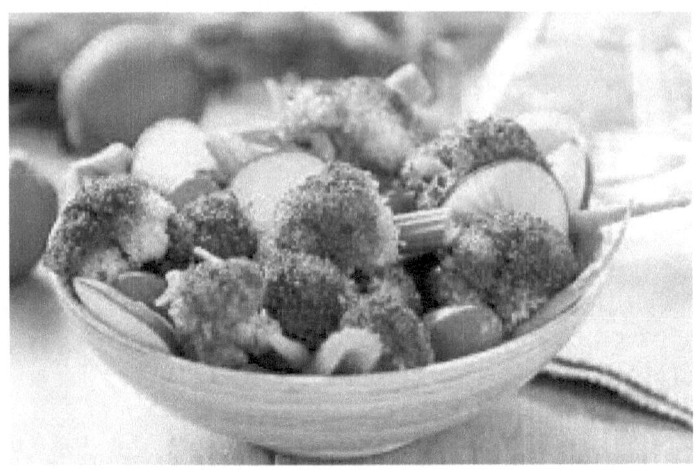

Does A Low Calorie Diet Work For Weight Loss?

In times past counting calories was the preferred recommendation for those of us trying to lose weight.

Every weight loss book, magazine and television show told us to follow a low calorie diet, eat low calorie meals and snacks but we don't hear it so often today so what happened?

It seems that today the hype is all about low carb, high protein diets but those in the know still maintain that a low calorie diet is still the best way to approach weight loss.

It seems that reducing our daily calorie intake is has been proven to still be the best way to reduce our waistlines but what constitutes a low calorie diet?

A general rule of thumb is that a low-cal diet is one in which the dieter consumes somewhere between 1000 and

1500 calories per day but it's important to realise that as we are all different and we all have different lifestyles, different energy expenditure and even different starting points a low calorie diet can be different for everyone.

For me, sitting at my desk all day writing weight loss articles, a low calorie diet might be measured at 1000 calories but for you, if you have a physically energetic job, [you're a bricklayer or a busy mother and housewife], 1500 calories might be nearer the mark.

A good healthy goal is to aim to lose about 1/2 to 1 kilo per week [that's 1-2 pounds] and when we first begin our low calorie diet we may well find that we'll lose more than that because in the initial stages we tend to lose more water.

We shouldn't get discouraged if, after a week or three our rate of weight loss slows down, it's only natural because it's harder for us to actually lose the fat than it is to lose water, perhaps it's as well to remember that slow progress towards our weight loss goals is still progress, we don't need to think that because we're only losing 1 kilo per week not thc 5 kilos we were losing initially that our low calorie diet is no longer working.

It's also very important to make sure that the food we're eating while we're on our diet is healthy and nutritious.

We need to ensure that we get enough protein each day to maintain our skin tone and muscle strength, lean meat, fish eggs, beans ctc. all have a high degree of protein and even on a low calorie diet we need to eat up to 100 grams of carbohydrates daily and 20 grams of fibre to help our digestion.

While we want to lose weight we should keep our fat intake down to below 30% of our total calorie intake and less than 25% of that fat should be saturated fats [butter, cheese, red meat and other animal-based foods] because medical science has proved that saturated fats can have a detrimental effect on our health by raising our "bad" cholesterol levels and increasing our risk of heart disease.

When we combine a low calorie diet with regular sensible exercise we will lose all the weight we need to lose without depriving ourselves of the good wholesome foods that our bodies need to function as they should.

One last point for this post, we shouldn't think of skipping meals in order to keep the calorie count down, it just doesn't work.

When we don't eat regular meals our metabolism slows down and we burn fat much more slowly, it's better to eat even a very small meal rather than no meal at all.

Regardless of our age, if we're over-weight and feel that we need to do something about it then a low calorie diet is a good way to go and if we're not sure how to go about it then a visit to the doctor or a licenced dietician will put us on the right track.

While we may not lose weight quickly with a low calorie diet with a little patience and some persistence we will ultimately lose all the weight we need to.

Diets that deliver food to your door, pre-packaged and ready to eat [except for heating] are called fixed menu diets.

With a fixed menu diet we will know exactly what we're going to eat for each meal every day because we purchase it in advance.

This is possibly the easiest diet to adhere to because it takes almost all the diet decision making away from us, the downside to this type of diet plan is that we don't learn how to make food decisions for ourselves and the food can be quite boring and tasteless.

Another drawback is it isn't easy to take ready packaged meals with us when we travel but, as a starting point for weight loss beginners a fixed menu diet is a reasonable place to start.

THE EXCHANGE DIET.

If we follow an exchange diet we choose our foods from the different food groups, for example we might choose pasta as our starch for this meal, potatoes as our starch for the next and so on.

An advantage to the exchange diet is that we can make our meals different each day, we get to choose what we eat and we learn to make good food choices.

THE FORMULA DIET.

When we put ourselves on a formula diet we will be drinking most of our meals in the form of shakes of one kind or another with only one meal each day consisting of "real food".

The shakes or liquid formulas are generally full of proteins and carbohydrates and contain little by way of either good or bad fats.

Formula diets are convenient, easy to follow, often inexpensive and will help us to lose weight in the short term however they can be difficult to continue in the long run.

THE ORNISH DIET.

The Ornish Diet is a little different to most diets we read about.

Most of us think of losing weight when we see the word "diet" and the Ornish Diet will help us to do that but its proponents say it can be adjusted to suit the circumstances and needs of those who follow it.

If we need to lose weight we can adjust it for that, if we would like to prevent or reverse diabetes for example, it can, apparently, help us there, if we need to lower our blood pressure or lower our cholesterol, well it's claimed to be of benefit there, there are even some who believe that it's useful for the prevention and treatment of breast and prostate cancer.

[Please don't rely on this, or any diet for the treatment of these very serious conditions, take advice from your healthcare professional].

We can change our eating habits a little if we only need to get little changes, lose just a kilo or two for example, or we can go the whole hog and make drastic adjustments if we need drastic results.

The Ornish Diet makes the claim that: "It's scientifically proven to make you feel better, live longer, lose weight and gain health."

RAW FOOD DIET.

Those who are fans of the Raw Food Diet tell us that raw food is jam packed with nutrients and natural enzymes that will help our bodies reach their best possible health and when we do that we will naturally lose weight.

Raw foods haven't been processed in any way, nor have they been treated with pesticides or preservatives and they include such things as nuts, fresh fruit, berries, vegetables, herbs and seeds.

Although there is no scientific evidence to support the belief, those who eat a raw food diet claim that cooking removes most of the goodness in what we eat, but scientifically what makes the raw food diet work is that those who follow it only consume about half the calories they would eat if they ate a cooked food diet.

Whichever type of diet we choose it is quite important to combine it with a reasonable amount of sensible exercise to ensure that our bodies are using the foods we eat in an efficient manner and to build our muscle tone, strength and flexibility.

Because of the sheer number of different diets and diet types which are promoted and the general confusion over which diets work and which diets don't it is generally recommended that we each consult with a weight loss professional, that's a dietician, nutritionist or medical professional, to determine which of the various diets will be best for each of us, that way we get the best information to suit our individual needs.

THE VEGAN DIET.

Vegans will tell us that taking meat and dairy products from our diet completely will inevitably lead to weight loss, and so it might.

It is also possible that "going Vegan" may help with our general health by reducing the danger that comes from heart disease, cancer and diabetes.

THE VOLUMETRICS DIET.

The theory of the volumetrics diet is that we all have a tendency to eat the same amount, or volume, of food regardless of how many calories it contains and therefore, according to its proponents, if we eat what is referred to as "less dense foods", that is foods with less calories, we will automatically lose weight.

Filling our plates with these "less dense" foods we should find that we can satisfy our hunger with a normal [for us] amount of food but consume fewer calories in doing so.

Filling up on vegetables and fruit is a preferred way to go as, for example, about 30 grams of peanuts contain as many calories as half a kilo of carrots but, as we all know, half a kilo of carrots would fill most of our stomachs to overflowing.

THE WORST DIETS/WEIGHT LOSS PROGRAMS.

PICK YOUR POISON

GRAPEFRUIT DIET   LOW CARB   3 DAY FAST   Volumetrics
Lemonade Diet   **3 DAY DIET**   LOW FAT   FRUIT FLUSH
BANANA DIET   CABBAGE SOUP DIET   The Werewolf Diet
3 DAY TUNA DIET   DASH DIET   Zone Diet   FAT FREE
Alkaline Diet   BABY FOOD DIET   South Beach   RAW FOOD DIET
The Cookie Diet   Five Bite Diet   Blood Type Diet
Sleeping Beauty Diet   HCG Diet   The Tapeworm Diet

What are the worst diets that we can try without the very real danger of causing ourselves perhaps permanent damage?

Of course, there are any number of bad diets we can find if we search for them, everybody and his uncle has a favourite weight loss programme or diet that they swear by.

"If you only drink cabbage water for ten days you'll lose all the weight you want"....."If you only eat every third day and only drink water on the other two you're going to lose umpteen kilos in a month".....

We've all seen them, most of us have firsthand experience from friends and relatives who, of course, only have our best interests at heart but what about the diets that are promoted on the internet or by celebrities who are trying to convince us that this or that diet is the real thing.

Perhaps the first thing we should understand is that there is no magical weight loss pill or supplement that will cause us to lose weight with little or no effort regardless of the celebrity hype that surrounds it.

Part of the diet conundrum is that almost all the diets and weight loss programs we try will initially cause us to lose weight but maintaining that initial weight loss is much more difficult and let's face it, losing weight only to put it back on again shortly afterwards does us no good at all.

What I have tried to do here is compile a short sampling of the types of bad diets that we see promoted that are, in fact, all but useless and which we should avoid if we don't want to be disappointed yet again.

FAD DIETS.

Fad diets of any description will fail in the longer term and may even cause us to regain more weight than we lose when we, inevitably, quit from deprivation and frustration.

Some examples of fad diets might be diets that focus on specific groups of food such as cabbage water, vegan only foods, raw food diets and very low carb diets.

We should be wary of any diet that suggests that we should avoid certain food groups altogether, our bodies are designed to consume a large variety of foodstuffs in order to get all of the nutrients which they need to function properly and restricting our consumption of certain foods normally just leads to us craving that which we have restricted.

DETOX DIETS.

Any diet that requires extreme methods like colonic cleansing, liver flushes, hormone injections etc. are very suspect, our bodies do not need to be "flushed", we have the necessary organs built in to do the job quite adequately.

Our liver and kidneys were designed for that very purpose and there is no scientific evidence to suggest that they need any help to do their job.

"MIRACLE" PILLS AND POTIONS.

As dieters most of us are looking for easier ways to lose weight and the promise of taking this pill twice a day or drinking this potion to replace a meal or two can look like an easy answer to our weight loss efforts.

We should realise, as I've said above, that there is no "miracle" weight loss pill, no magic potion which will make us lose weight, indeed no single food, either eaten on its own or in combination with others or eaten in a specific way or at a certain time of day will help us to lose weight one little bit.

Expensive supplements are just that, expensive and totally unnecessary.

FASTING.

Fasting is fine perhaps as a religious exercise or on doctors orders but fasting to lose weight is counter-productive.

If we don't consume all the calories we need our bodies tend to think they are actually starving and so our metabolism slows down.

When we revert to our normal eating habits, as surely we will, our metabolism doesn't re-adjust, we need fewer calories than we did but we're back to our original calorie intake hence we put on weight.

This particular pattern is called "the yoyo syndrome" or "weight cycling", we lose weight, we put it back on, we lose weight, we put it back on, and so on.

VERY LOW CALORIE DIETS.

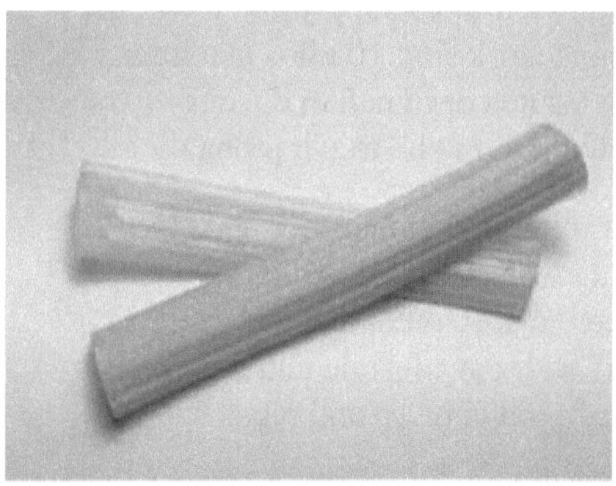

Any diet we hear about that promises dramatic weight loss in very short periods of time, such as most very low cal diets, are completely unrealistic.

With very low calorie diets we may experience some initial weight loss but most, if not all of that will be water and the possible side effects from a very low calorie diet may be things like extreme tiredness, diarrhoea, nausea and constipation or more commonly the formation of gallstones which are very uncomfortable and can also be very serious.

TOO GOOD TO BE TRUE DIETS.

We've all heard the saying " if it sounds too good to be true it probably is' and this applies to our weight loss efforts just as everywhere else in life.

The email that tells us that the sender has finally found the "secret" to easy weight loss: "PSSST don't tell anyone else about this, there's only a limited supply and it will be gone soon" and the promise of losing 10 kilos in a week sounds very convincing, as it is designed to do, but remember, if it sounds too good to be true it probably is.

When searching for a weight loss strategy for ourselves we need to realise that there is no "one size fits all" weight loss plan, we need to seek out a diet and exercise plan that, first of all, fits with our lifestyle and focuses on healthier, better balanced food choices and regular, moderate exercise.

When we do that we'll find that we can lose weight, keep it off and feel, and be better for it.

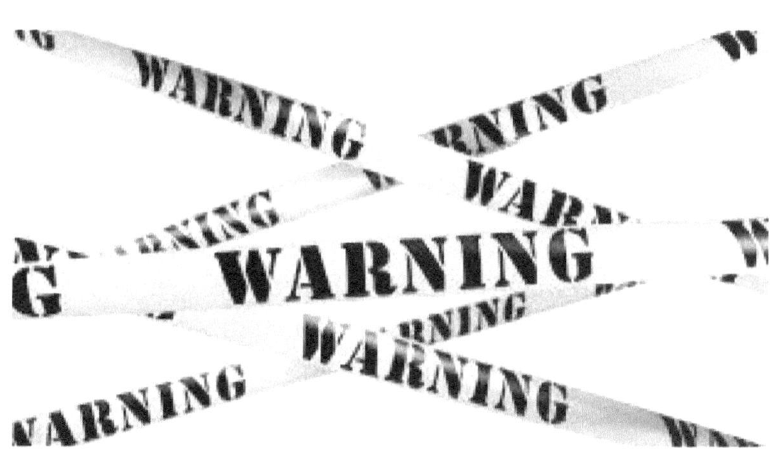

Everybody who has ever had a weight problem has, at one time or another tried to diet the weight away.

We've all done it and almost without exception we've all had at least one failed attempt to lose weight this way and while there are some good diet programs available there is also an awful lot of rubbish, fad diets, and dangerous weight loss programs, much of it promoted on the internet, and a great deal of it just downright dangerous.

I can't write about all the dangerous fad diets and programs on this page but I can give us some insights as to what to avoid when considering a plan in our own effort to lose weight.

Here are some things we need to be careful of when deciding to diet our way to weight loss.

VERY LOW CALORIE DIETS, LONG TERM FASTING, STARVATION DIETS.

When we put ourselves through the rigours of Very Low Calorie Diets, Long Term Fasting or Starvation Diets we will certainly lose weight, especially if we stick to it for a while however the weight we lose will include a significant percentage of muscle which, in turn, will lower our metabolism and cause our body to retain a higher percentage of fat thereby increasing the chances of developing type 2 diabetes amongst other conditions.

We'll find in our research references to the ABC Diet, also known as "Anorexics Boot Camp" which is just this type of "starvation" diet, very dangerous and to be avoided at all costs.

Anorexia is an illness not a diet and it's a very serious illness at that, not to be messed with as it can cause all manner of permanent damage to our bodies.

No-one with any sense at all wants to risk things like a heart attack, a brain shutdown or colossal failure of the liver or the pancreas or the stomach just to lose a few kilos.

This is one fad "diet" which is extremely dangerous.

THE K-E DIET.

The K-E Diet, more properly known as the Ketogenic Enternal Nutrition diet or feeding tube diet is a dangerous fad diet during which the dieter does not eat or drink for a period of 10 days but instead is "fed" through a tube inserted via the nostril.

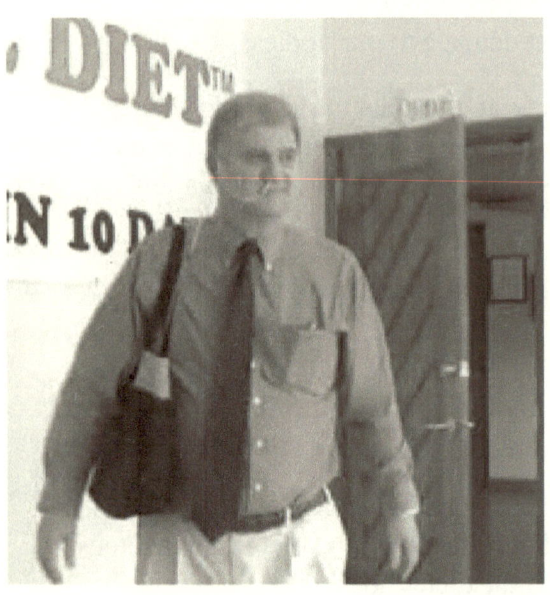

Very popular with brides to be in some countries the feeding tube diet apparently does cause some rapid weight loss, as, I guess, you would expect from not eating for 10 days, but apart from the inconvenience of having to carry a bag of fluid around with you 24/7 with a tube stuck up your nose there are some very real health risks associated with this fad diet.

The least of these health concerns may be things like bad breath, lack of energy and some bad constipation, the more serious may cause kidney failure, the possibility of infection caused by sticking a tube up your nose and potential future eating disorders as your body decides it's easier to get its food this way.

As fad diets got the feeding tube diet is one to definitely stay away from.

We've heard it before from any number of sources about all sorts of things, 11 little words that we all need to take notice of.

"If it sounds too good to be true, it probably is."

Companies that make prescription drugs have to prove that they work and that they are safe to take.

They must satisfy the relevant authorities that their products are effective for doing the job that they are being advertised to do.

For example, if you take a tablet to control diabetes the company that manufacture that drug must put it through rigorous testing to prove to the governments of the world that it will control diabetes as stated on the packaging and won't cause any major or unknown side effects.

Not so with weight loss supplements.

The manufacturers of these weight loss supplements don't have to prove anything to anybody before they can sell you their product.

Another thing to be wary of is the claim that the product is "all natural" or contains nothing artificial, this doesn't make it safe to take or effective for controlling our weight.

After all, if we think about it there are a zillion things that occur naturally in this world that will kill us almost instantly.

Just remember: "If it sounds too good to be true, it probably is."

PURGING.

One very good definition of purging as found in most good dictionaries is "to clear or empty (the bowels) by causing evacuation."

Making ourselves vomit after eating, over using laxatives to empty our bowels and chewing food but not actually swallowing it are all behaviours which are associated with purging.

These purging behaviours are not uncommon amongst young women in particular, can pose some very serious health risks and are often the beginning to the development of unhealthy eating disorders such as anorexia and bulimia.

Also associated with purging could be the damage caused by the regurgitation of our very strong stomach acid, burning the throat and mouth and causing some tooth decay if we do it often.

Purging by induced vomiting or the use of strong laxatives is no way to lose weight, it's just not worth it.

OVER EXERCISING.

Over exercising is worth a mention here.

When you watch some of the "reality" shows on
television and you see obese people being encouraged to
exercise to their absolute limits it's important to realise
first of all that they are doing so to make "good"
television and secondly that they are very well
supervised.

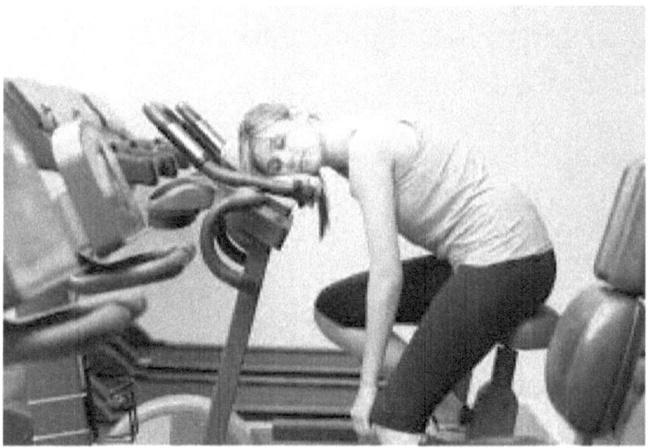

In the real world, that's the world that you and I live in,
extreme exercising is not only foolish but extreme
exercise can be extremely dangerous.

When we push our bodies to do things which they are not
accustomed to doing we increase the opportunity for us
to injure ourselves, often severely, we increase the
amount of wear on our joints, we probably add extra
strain to our tendons and ligaments and we risk things
like dehydration and so on.

There are also psychological implications such as
thinking of exercise as punishing ourselves for over
eating.

A healthy weight loss programme does include exercise but it's healthy exercise as recommended by our relevant health professionals such as our dietician, our medical doctor and our qualified personal trainer.

Becoming obsessed with extreme exercise is counterproductive in the long run, is unlikely to become a permanent part of our weight loss regime and may cause us more harm than good.

WEIGHT LOSS DRUGS.

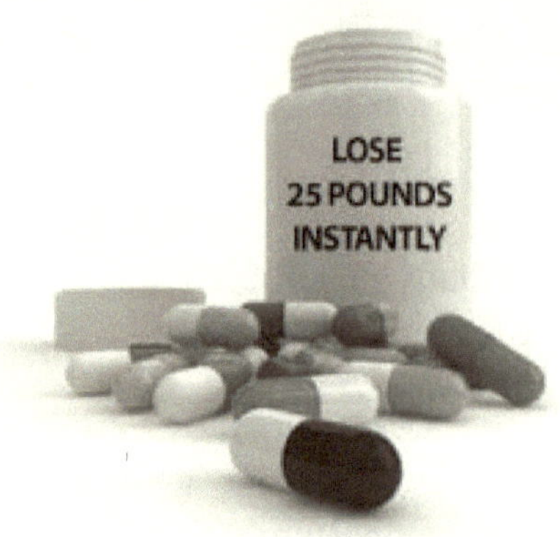

Again worth mentioning, taking weight loss drugs which are not prescribed by our health professionals can, and often do, have very serious consequences.

The potential damage which we can suffer by using such things as cigarettes as a substitute for food in order to lose weight is incalculable and taking drugs which have been prescribed for some other condition is risking severe problems with our health, both physical and mental.

The bottom line here is be sensible, if we need to use weight loss drugs to help us with our weight loss make sure we get them prescribed for us for that specific purpose.

As I said earlier there are too many dangerous/fad diets for me to mention here but if we are wise and listen to the voice of reason which we all have we can avoid those things which will do us more harm than good and we can lose all the weight we want to lose in a safe and healthy way.

Do yourself a favour and check with your medical professional before embarking on any weight loss diet, it is the only sensible thing to do.

CRASH DIETS.

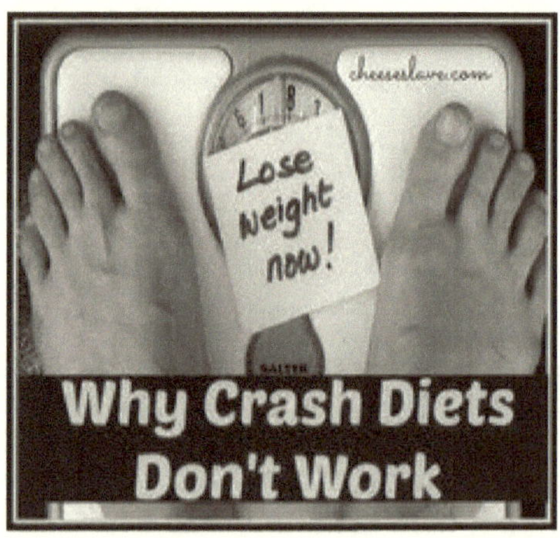

Do Crash Diets Make Us Fatter?

Like it or not we live in an instant world, everything happens so quickly.

Today we can send a letter to someone on the other side of the globe and they receive it within milliseconds, we can make a cup of coffee in the time it takes to boil some water we can even travel from A to B, regardless of where A and B are, in so little time it's almost scary, so why can't we lose weight just as instantly?

The question that gets asked most often of dieticians and personal trainers is not "how can I lose weight?" but "how can I lose weight quickly?"

Whether we're going on holiday, getting married or just need to lose a few kilos for another special event we all seem to want to do it in as short a time as possible.

That is often where our weight loss efforts start to go off track because while it is definitely possible to lose weight quickly it's neither healthy nor permanent when we do.

Gaining weight is often a process that takes some time; many of us have seen just a small increase in our waistlines and therefore our weight over a period of many years.

Twenty years ago I weighed 80 kilos, fifteen years ago it was 83 kilos, ten years ago it was 88 kilos and I'll bet that your story it not too much different to that.

Weight gain seems often to creep up on us and it's only when we have to prepare for that special occasion or perhaps we have a medical wakeup call or look in the mirror one day and realise we've become what we always vowed we would never be, too big for our pants or skirts, that we decide that we need to lose, [sometimes a lot of] weight and we want to do it *NOW!*

It's at this point that many of us will turn to one of the many "quick fix" crash diets which are available today.

We can find crash diets anywhere, they're promoted in the local pharmacy, in every woman's magazine and a search on Google for "lose weight quickly" will return almost 25 million results, but will a crash diet actually work for us?

Sadly, as many have discovered, the answer is "no".

The reason for this sad state of affairs is that when we embark on a crash diet we are essentially changing our metabolism.

An extremely low calorie diet, which most crash diets are, will very effectively slow our metabolism because when we restrict our intake of energy producing foods our bodies will compensate for that lack of energy by slowing down.

This is just one of the many reasons very obese people struggle so much when trying to lose weight.

The many cleansing, detoxing, very restrictive crash diet plans available are, in fact, doing us more harm than good.

Many of us have heard of, if not watched "the biggest loser", a weight loss television show, and perhaps marvelled at the results some of the contestants get but a

recent study
[http://coach.nine.com.au/2016/05/03/10/17/biggest-
loser-contestants-have-slow-metabolisms] has shown
that when they leave the show their bodies often never
recover from the extremes of diet and exercise they were
subjected to.

The study found that a severe diet and exercise regime
slows a body's metabolism to such an extent that it loses
the ability to bounce back, effectively meaning that after
such a drastic weight loss program we have to continue
to severely restrict our calorie intake in order to maintain
the weight loss.

In practical terms the result is that when we remove the
severe restrictions of our crash diets and begin to eat
"normally" again we will put on more weight than we
lost in the first place.

Generally we put weight on slowly and if we need to lose
weight that should also be a controlled, and yes, a
relatively slow process.

Rapid weight loss is possible but it definitely isn't the
best way to lose weight nor is it healthy or permanent.

Drinking nothing but cabbage water for a week or two
will undoubtedly make us lose weight, not because we
are "cleansing" our bodies of toxins but because we're
consuming next to no calories [and spending too much
time on the toilet].

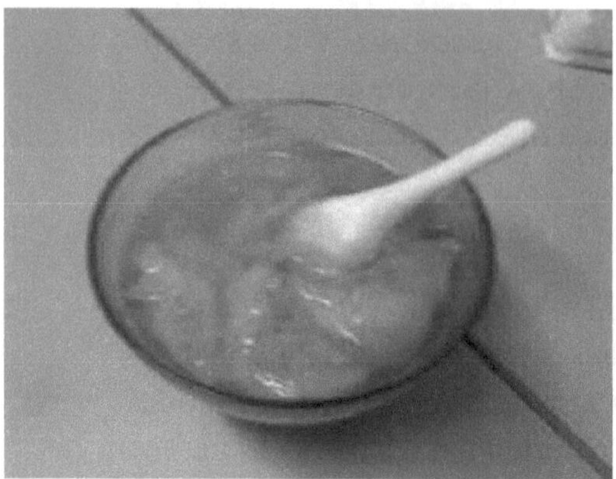

When we think that it's probably taken many years for us to put on the weight is it unreasonable to expect that it may take just a little time to lose the weight we've managed to accumulate?

The best way to lose weight is to do it with a reasonable diet and exercise program, stick at it without getting discouraged, don't beat yourself up if you go backwards every once in a while and in less time than you might imagine you'll begin to lose that weight and you'll be able to keep it off without stressing your body and causing yourself some very nasty health problems.

WHY IS MY DIET NOT WORKING?

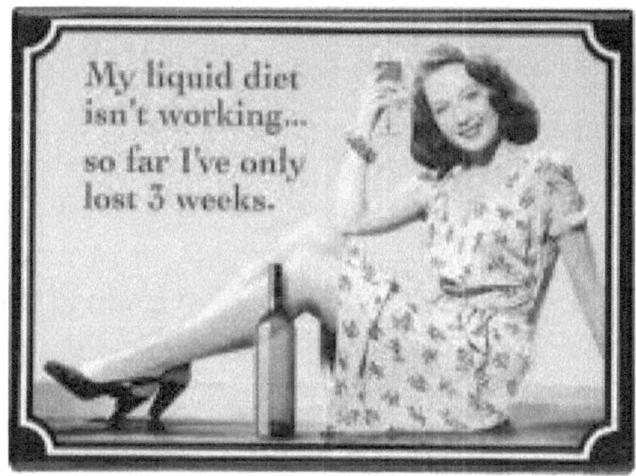

It's a question many of us have asked, sometimes multiple times.

After all, we've made the effort to stop eating those delicious sweet desserts, we haven't had a coke for so long we've gotten over the withdrawal symptoms and our portion sizes are "only half of what they used to be" but we still don't seem to be making any progress towards our weight loss goals.

Even an hour a day doing some form of energetic exercise isn't helping.

We're doing all the right things but it seems that we're just treading water, getting nowhere in our efforts to lose weight.

We ask ourselves again, why?

Often the answer to that question is that it is entirely possible that we've become bogged down in a dieting rut, we don't know what to do to escape from it and as a result we become frustrated and a bit depressed about our whole attempt to lose weight.

This frequently results in us eating to overcome the depression and when we do we tend to eat all the wrong things in all the wrong quantities and often we do it too many times.

The obvious result of this binge eating is that we undo all the previous weight loss gains we have made which, in turn, leaves us feeling guilty which makes us depressed and ......

You know the story.

Also many of us don't have the support systems in place to help us deal with these inevitable feelings of failure and our loved ones may not be helping if they don't, for example, make the effort to keep the fridge free of junk food or they eat things in front of us which we're trying to avoid.

It's not that they don't care it's more that they don't think about the struggle we are going through in our efforts to lose weight, a gentle hint should work.

When we're in this situation and nothing seems to be working for us it's a good idea to seek out some professional help by visiting a health professional who specialises in weight related issues.

A dietician is a good place to start, he or she will put us back on the right track and reinforce to us the steps we need to take to regain control of our weight loss efforts.

If we find that perhaps we've gone beyond the help of our dietician, if we've started to take extreme measures like binge eating and then purging or perhaps not eating at all then we need to face the probability that we need some psychotherapy to get us back on track.

There's no shame in seeking the appropriate help, it's the sensible thing to do when we're unable to fix things ourselves and it can only do good in the long run.

Another possible reason for our inability to lose weight could be that unknowingly we are consuming "hidden" calories.

The cappuccino which we love and have with our breakfast each morning and the frappuccino we have when we have lunch at Starbucks are loaded with calories, perhaps we should have them made with skim milk and we all know the soda we all love when we're thirsty is also loaded with calories.

Many of us have fallen into the trap of thinking that if we substitute "diet" soda for the "real" stuff it must surely help us in our weight loss efforts.

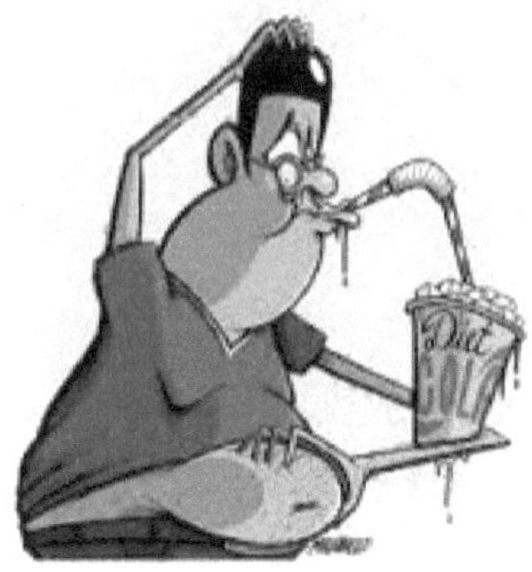

Not so!

Not only is any soda, diet or otherwise, very unhealthy in so many ways, scientific research has shown that when we substitute artificial sweeteners such as those in diet soda for the real thing our bodies recognise that we're not getting the calories we thought we would get, our metabolism gets out of whack and therefore our appetite increases and we eat more.

Finally for this post, a lack of consistency in our weight loss regime is another very real reason for a lack of progress towards our weight loss goals.

I've found it's easy to stick to a diet for a few days, sometimes even for a week or two but over time I tend to become complacent, I see the start of some real weight loss and I start to slip back into old habits, old ways of eating and bad diet choices.

I didn't really see any substantial weight loss progress until I stopped looking at my effort as "a diet" and started seeing it as a lifestyle change.

Now my "diet" has become a way of life, no longer something to be endured but rather something to be embraced and enjoyed.

Was it easy? No.

Was it worth it? Definitely.

Can we all do it? With a positive attitude and perhaps a little help along the way, yes we can and we'll all feel so much better for it.

Start today and look forward to the rest of your life with a new body and the new found freedom that comes with that.

NATURAL WEIGHT LOSS REMEDIES AND SUPPLEMENTS.

There are so many "natural" weight loss remedies and supplements available, and they're spruiked almost everywhere, that we might be forgiven if we think that just because they're supposedly natural and obviously popular they might just be an answer to our weight loss woes.

If this is you, think again.

As you probably already know, there is no "miracle cure" to the problem of being overweight or obese, it's a difficult condition which, for many of us is the result of a lifetime of wrong choices as far as our food and drink consumption is concerned.

Changing our diet and the eating habits we've come to enjoy isn't easy and actually getting out of the house to get some regular and worthwhile exercise just doesn't seem to be very appealing when it's difficult to just walk up the stairs so it becomes much easier to look for an answer which requires little effort on our part.

So, let's look at some of the more popular "natural" weight loss supplements which we can find on the shelves of any chemist in almost any country in the world.

5-HYDROXYTRYPTOPHAN (5-HTP).

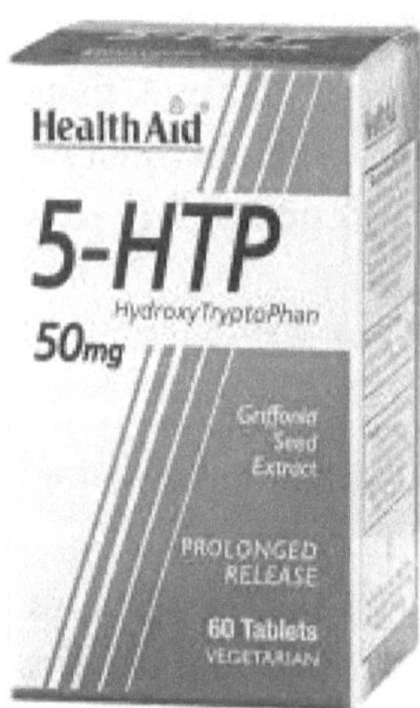

5-hydroxytryptophan (5-HTP) is another "natural" weight loss remedy which has a questionable record as far as effectiveness and safety is concerned.

Used as a replacement for Tryptophan weight loss supplements, many of which have been banned because they have the potential to cause some very unpleasant and possibly dangerous side effects, 5-HTP when taken causes our bodies to increase the production of serotonin which in turn helps our nerves and brains to work as they should.

Those who are advocates of 5-HTP claim that it suppresses the appetite and therefore aids weight loss and some initial trials seem to support this view however if we take large amounts of 5-HTP we may find the side effects such as an increase in headaches, nausea, muscle pain, anxiety and sleepiness far outweigh the possible weight loss benefits.

ALOE.

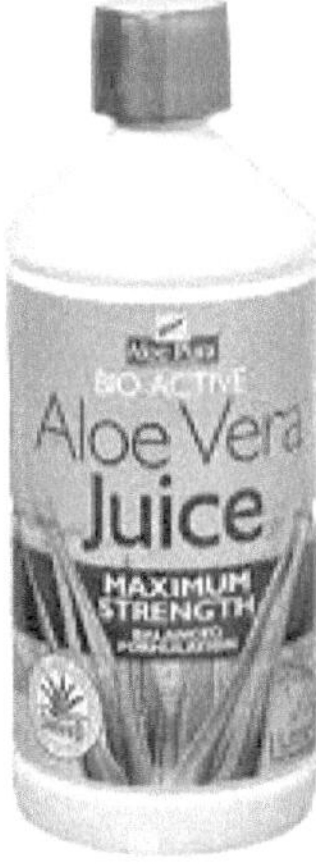

Aloe is a plant which has over 400 different varieties and when we think of Aloe we generally think of it as something we use as a salve on burns, cuts and abrasions and the like but Aloe is also added to many over the counter weight loss products because Aloe will clean our insides as well as our skin.

The most widely recognised species of Aloe is Aloe Vera which is claimed to have great medicinal properties and is included by many cosmetic companies for its skin rejuvenating effects and although Aloe has been promoted by many as a cure for all sorts of ailments it seems that the only thing it will actually fix is constipation because Aloe is a proven laxative.

The scientific studies indicate that Aloe has absolutely no reason to be included in weight loss products as it provides no weight loss benefits except, of course, the weight loss we'll experience from the side effects of taking Aloe which include strong bowel movements, abdominal cramping, diarrhoea and the disturbance of the natural vitamin balance in our bodies.

Possibly the one worthwhile thing Aloe has going for it when taken internally is that it contains a high degree of collagen protein which means that including it in our diet could increase our protein intake but, for me, the side effects are just not worth the supposed benefits.

AYURVEDA.

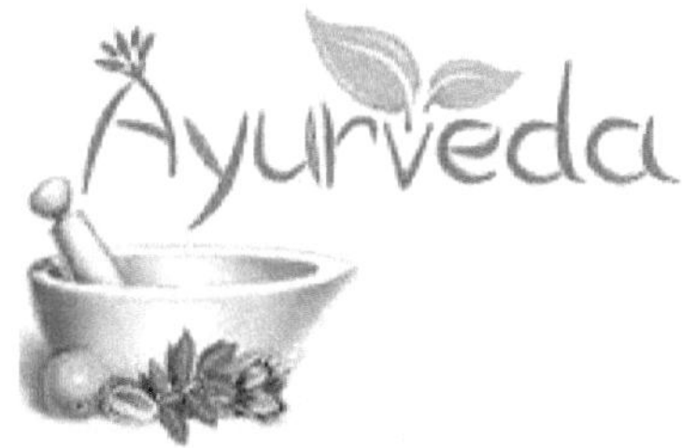

Ayurveda is not a weight loss supplement but it is more a [very] beneficial way of life and weight loss, or attaining the correct weight for each of us, is a by-product of that.

The over-riding belief behind Ayurveda is that excess weight comes from over-eating, incorrect eating habits and an unbalanced diet and in order to correct that Ayurveda devotees recommend an easy to follow diet which consists of greater portions of fruit and vegies while reducing the intake of salt, dairy products rich in fat and meat.

There is much more to the practice of Ayurveda, way too much for me to consider here but it seems to be a possible answer to many of life's uncomfortable situations including obesity, if you'd like to find out more I recommend Dr. Deepak Chopra's Ayurveda page.

[http://www.chopra.com/articles/what-is-ayurveda]

BITTER ORANGE/ SYNEPHRINE.

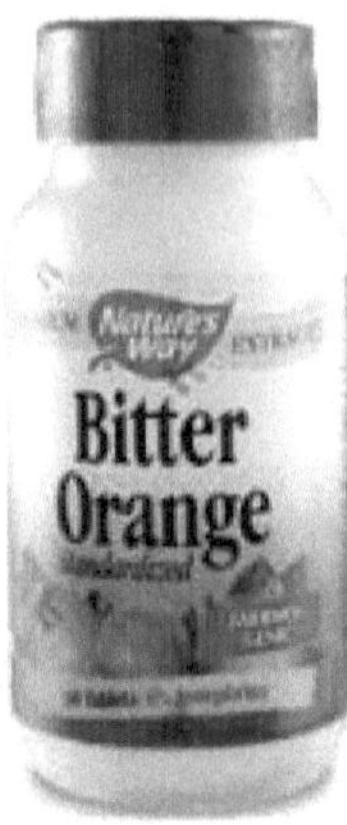

Bitter Orange, also known by many other names, is often used in weight loss supplements as a substitute for Ephedra which has been banned in many countries as being unsafe.

Natural weight loss supplements which are advertised as "Ephedra free" often contain Bitter Orange which has an almost identical chemical formula to Ephedra and is likely to be just as unsafe.

Containing octopamine and synephrine, both chemicals which are proven to cause high blood pressure and heart problems, Bitter Orange is a natural weight loss supplement which should be viewed with extreme caution and never, ever taken without first consulting a medical doctor.

As well as the obvious health risks associated with Bitter Orange there is some reliable evidence that it may interfere with our bodies ability to metabolise many other legitimate drugs we may need to take thereby adding another level of potential danger to our health.

With no dependable scientific study to determine the efficiency of Bitter Orange as a natural weight loss supplement we would be best advised to leave it on the shelf whenever we find it.

CAFFEINE.

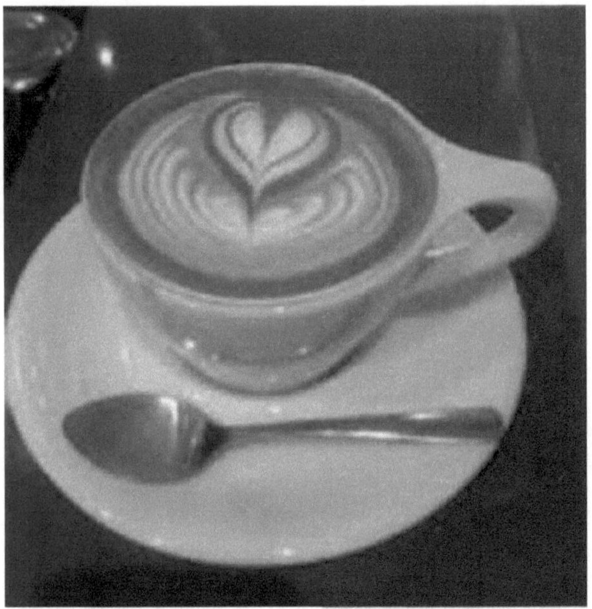

Well known as the world's most popular, and therefore the most consumed mood enhancer, caffeine is found naturally in coffee [you didn't know that?], green tea and dark chocolate and is added to countless manufactured foods and drinks.

Caffeine is also a staple in many commercial weight loss products for its metabolism boosting effects as a number of small scientific studies have indicated that caffeine may boost our metabolism by as much as 11% and increase the amount of fat we burn by up to 29%.

On the down side caffeine can have some very irritating if not hugely dangerous side effects for those of us who are affected by it.

As well as the well documented insomnia caffeine can also cause us to become jittery and irritable, give us nausea and diarrhoea and other symptoms.

At the end of the day there really is no need to take a weight loss supplement with caffeine in it, all we need to do is drink more coffee [and eat more dark chocolate?].

CASCARA.

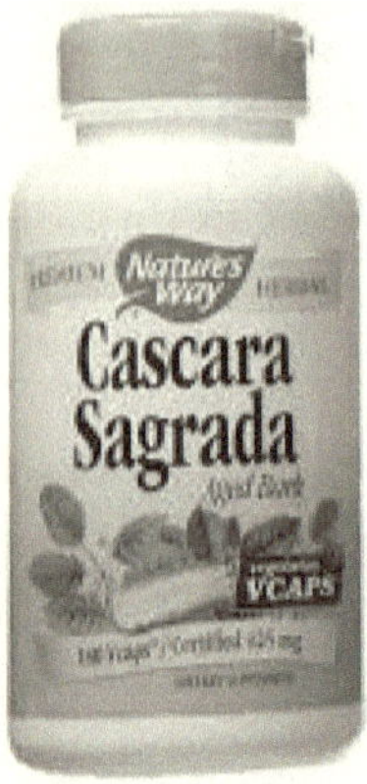

Cascara is the generally accepted term for a substance found in any number of "natural" weight loss supplements.

Previously approved by the US Food and Drug Administration (FDA), Cascara, or to give it its more formal title Cascara Sagrada, could be purchased as an over the counter drug for the treatment for constipation but since late 2002 it has been prohibited for sale as a drug due to concerns about the side effects on our health, this however hasn't stopped it's sale as a weight loss supplement as weight loss supplements are not required to undergo any formal government testing or approval.

Because of its very strong laxative effects the use of Cascara will provide short term weight loss but it should be used with extreme caution and should never be taken for more than 14 days or if you're pregnant or breast-feeding or if you have any gastro-intestinal problems.

Cascara is one of those preparations which MAY have some benefits but should be taken only after obtaining the proper advice.

CHITOSAN.

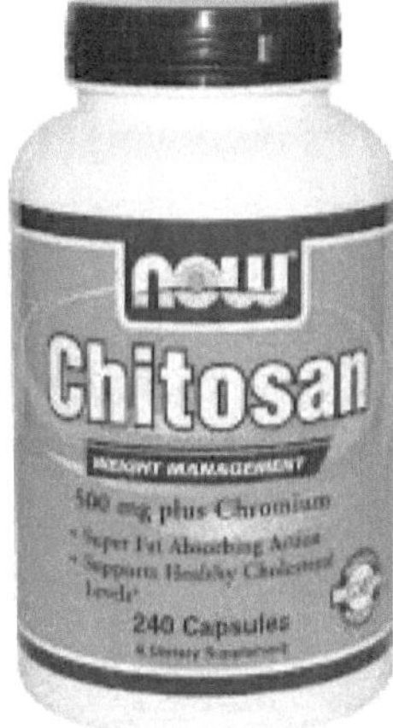

Chitosan is a weight loss supplement which is made from the hard shell of various crustaceans such as crabs, prawns and the like and it has been used as a treatment for many ailments for many years.

As well as a multi-purpose "cure-all" it is also used to clarify wine, to prevent fungal infections in plants, it is used as a blood clotting agent in wound dressings, is hypoallergenic and has natural anti-bacterial properties.

But what about Chitosan as a weight loss supplement, does it work?

Well the short answer seems to be.........Maybe!

The theory is that Chitosan is a natural fat attractor and is sold as a natural weight loss supplement on the claim that it attracts the excess fat from our bodies and expels it in the normal way.

Some trials of Chitosan seem to indicate that in its natural state it may remove about 30-40 calories each day from our diet, and when modified, such as how we purchase it from our weight loss supplement supplier it is claimed to absorb three to five times its own weight in oil and fat.

The aforementioned trials were, as far as I can tell, performed on animals not people and even there the results are inconclusive, what is evident however is that most professionals in the weight loss industry agree that, as a weight loss supplement Chitosan doesn't do the job.

Try it by all means as it appears to have many good health benefits including as a treatment for high cholesterol, Crohn's disease and so on but be aware, if you're allergic to shellfish stay away from it and, as always, before you try any weight loss supplements or weight loss pills consult with your medical professional.

CHROMIUM.

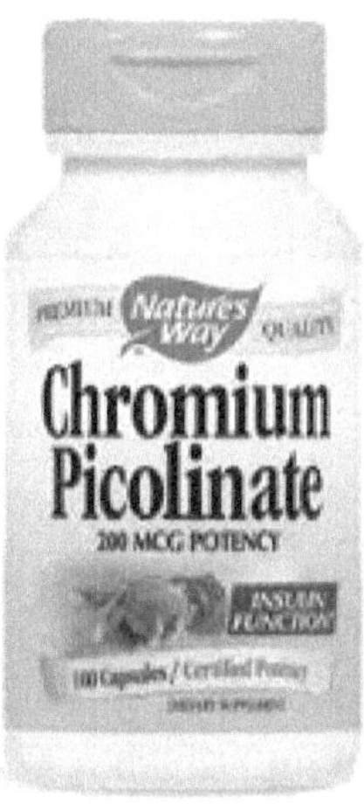

Chromium Picolinate, also known as just plain Chromium, is actually a chemical compound made up of chromium and picolinic acid and while Chromium itself is a necessary part of a healthy diet, our bodies need very small amounts of chromium and this can be found in sufficient quantities in fresh fruit and vegetables, whole grains and meat, the products which are promoted as "containing Chromium Picolinate" for weight loss are actually as good as useless.

A very popular "weight loss remedy" Chromium Picolinate is also touted as being useful in melting fat, reducing appetite and boosting the metabolism, claims which are dubious to say the least.

It reads like a dieters dream product on the label especially when you add the even more dubious claim that it increases lean muscle mass and improves our strength.

We can find Chromium Picolinate everywhere we look for weight loss supplements but with a plethora of possible side effects and absolutely no scientific evidence to support the claims of its promoters Chromium

Picolinate is another of the "natural weight loss supplements" we would probably be better off without.

CITRICOMA.

Relatively new to the ever increasing list of natural weight loss supplements, Citricoma is marketed by the makers of Cortislim which has been available since 2003.

Citricoma is apparently a blend of citrus polymethoxylated flavones [which are natural antioxidants and are used for the treatment of high cholesterol, varicose veins, cataracts, heart disease, and cancer] and Eurycoma longifolia which is a plant found in South East Asia and the root of which is used in that part of the world for treating such things as erectile dysfunction, malaria, high blood pressure, syphilis and any number of other medical conditions.

While the jury is still out on the weight loss benefits of Citricoma if we read the various reports it seems it may be effective as a weight loss supplement as well as being quite beneficial to our health in other ways.

Citricoma may, repeat may, help to maintain normal levels of testosterone which is important during times of weight loss, it may reduce our cholesterol levels and the Eurycoma may help us to avoid the "dieters yo-yo" where we tend to lose weight only to put it back on in a never ending cycle.

Will Citricoma help us to lose weight? I don't know the answer to that however it looks promising and is probably worth trying but, as always, we should consult our doctor before we do to make sure it won't interfere with any other medications we're taking.

CONJUGATED LINOLEIC ACID (CLA).

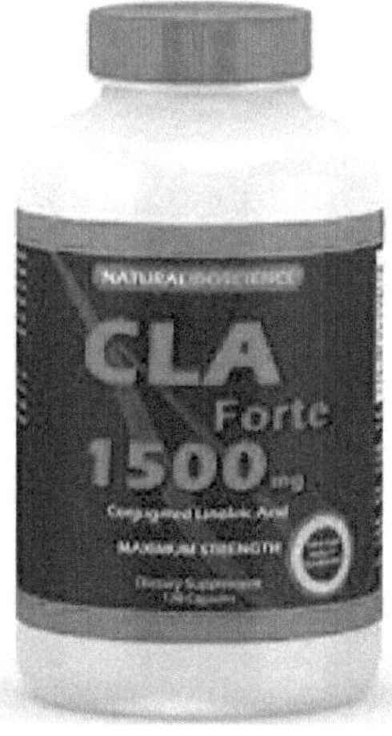

Conjugated Linoleic Acid has been around as a weight loss supplement for more years than I care to remember, first found in 1987 and explored as a possible cancer fighting agent it's now promoted as a healthy trans fat and is found to occur naturally in some everyday fatty foods such as beef and many dairy products.

It has been proven in a number of scientific studies to actually work in helping with our weight loss especially when combined with a healthy diet and reasonable exercise.

It should be noted however that the Conjugated Linoleic Acid which is found in weight loss supplements is not the naturally occurring CLA but is actually manufactured by a chemical process which alters the makeup up of sunflower and safflower oils which are, in fact, unhealthy vegetable oils.

The CLA weight loss supplements have been shown to cause some weight loss but the effects are so small and the trials so inconclusive that supplements containing CLA are probably not going to help us in the long run.

If we want to get the weight loss benefits of Conjugated Linoleic Acid we must consume more of the foods that contain it in its natural form.

DANDELION.

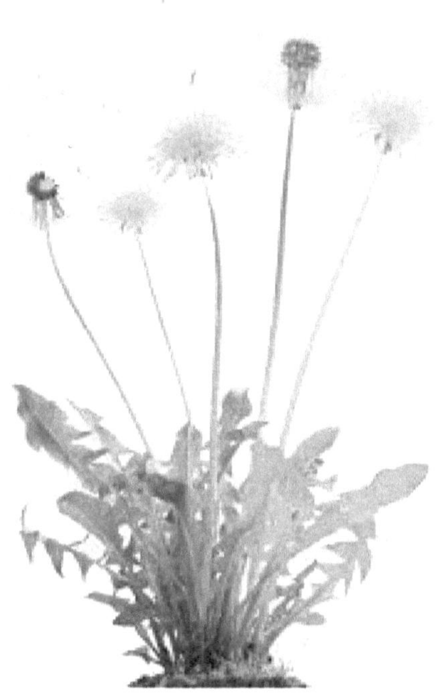

Dandelion, apart from being the plant that many of us curse when we see it spring up and spoil our lawns has a surprising number of beneficial uses [and a surprising number of pseudonyms].

Dandelion leaves can be used as part of our salads or raw on sandwiches, the roots of the dandelion make an acceptable substitute for coffee and the flower is used to make wine and schnapps.

Over the years, in various parts of the world the humble dandelion has been used for medicinal purposes to treat such things as boils, fever, diarrhoea, skin disorders, digestive problems and so on and being a natural diuretic dandelion may cause some weight loss purely from the action of decreasing the amount of fluid our bodies retain.

This being said, dandelion may also cause severe allergic reaction and heartburn so should be taken with caution.

Dandelion has been used for a lot of years and so has a history to support many, but not all, of the claims made by those who promote it.

Perhaps some of the more questionable claims include the effect it may have in flushing toxins from our systems, that it will boost our metabolism and also that it will reduce our cravings for sweets, but it should be noted that prolonged consumption of dandelion leaves or dandelion tea may cause dehydration and an imbalance of our electrolytes due to its diuretic effects.

Dandelion, as with all other "natural" weight loss supplements, or weight loss supplements in general should be investigated thoroughly and discussed with our doctors before deciding to use it.

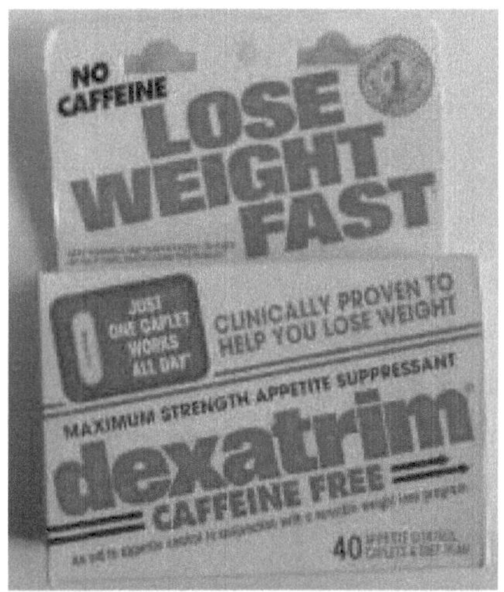

If you've been on the weight loss roundabout for any length of time you will already have come across Dexatrim in one of its many reincarnations and perhaps more than once.

Originally marketed in the 1970s Dexatrim has been taken off the market by the relevant authorities a number of times due to its links with various health issues however we can still buy it online and over the counter as an energy booster in the form of capsules or as an energy drink.

The Dexatrim website claims it is useful to boost energy, reduce stress, for appetite control and to fight fatigue but what are the facts behind the current formulations of Dexatrim?

It seems that the main ingredient in Dexatrim today is bitter orange peel which is used in the weight loss industry to replace the now banned Ephedra and it's mixed with several other so called "weight loss herbs" such as green tea, ginseng root, oolong tea and caffeine to make up the formulation.

There are several different formulations of Dexatrim depending on the outcome we're trying to achieve, they all have a slightly different make-up but they also all have some well documented, not very pleasant and perhaps dangerous side effects such as sleeplessness, jitteriness, nervousness, anxiety, irritability, upset stomach and nausea.

As a "natural" weight loss supplement Dexatrim offers little to help us to achieve our weight loss goals with the only real ingredient which may help us in that area being green tea extract and let's be sensible, we can buy green tea in any grocery store and get the benefits of it for just a few cents.

It's also interesting to note that hidden away at the bottom of each of the Dexatrim web pages is the following statement:

"STATEMENTS ON THIS SITE HAVE NOT BEEN EVALUATED BY THE FOOD AND DRUG ADMINISTRATION (FDA). PRODUCTS LISTED ARE NOT INTENDED TO DIAGNOSE, TREAT, CURE, OR PREVENT ANY DISEASE."

Ephedra has been used in traditional medicine in different countries for many years and has more recently been the main ingredient in a number of over the counter weight loss supplements.

As its main claim to fame, Ephedra was touted as an appetite suppressant which would cause us to feel less hungry and therefore eat less.

At first glance this would seem to be a reasonable supposition, after all, if we eat less we must surely lose weight mustn't we?

However not only has Ephedra been seen to have absolutely no effect when it comes to weight loss it has been scientifically proven to endanger the health of anyone who uses it, so much so that it has been banned in any of its forms from sale in the USA and other countries.

Ephedra is a proven stimulant and thermogenic and while the thermogenic properties should cause us to have an increase our metabolism and therefore burn off body fat the stimulant properties stimulates our brain, causes an increase in our heart rate and our blood pressure and causes an expansion in our bronchial passages.

The bottom line here is that while we may still be able to get weight loss supplements containing Ephedra from various sources it hasn't been banned for no reason, Ephedra and the weight loss pills containing it could very well end up killing those silly enough to take it.

FORSKOLIN.

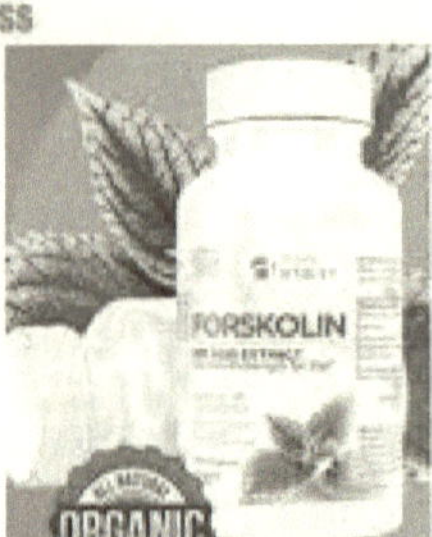

Forskolin is basically manufactured from the root of a mint plant that grows in South East Asia and has long been used as an ingredient in the traditional medicine of the region.

There is some belief that it contains a substance which stimulates the way our bodies burn fat and in very limited studies on men it has shown Forskolin reduced body fat and increased muscle mass but had no effect on weight.

Other studies show that it has no effect on women.

Supplements containing Forskolin have been taken for many reasons but there is little or no evidence to suggest that it has any beneficial effects either on our health or as a weight loss supplement.

The answer, as far as Forskolin is concerned, is that we would be better off avoiding it until some decent scientific studies have been undertaken.

GARCINIA CAMBOGIA EXTRACT.

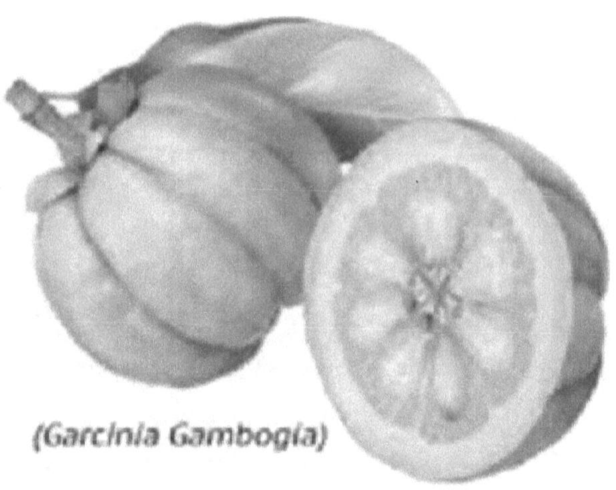

Possibly the most popular weight loss supplement currently available after it was shown on the Dr. Oz television programme in 2012, Garcinia Cambogia Extract with the active ingredient hydroxycitric acid (HCA) is derived from the skin of the Garcinia Cambogia plant which is a small green fruit that resembles a small pumpkin.

Garcinia Cambogia Extract "works" by supposedly inhibiting the production of fat in the body and by reducing food cravings.

Small studies have been carried out and the results suggest that there is no advantage to using Garcinia Cambogia Extract as opposed to a placebo and while there appear to be no major side effects some participants have experienced mild stomach problems.

Is HCA safe to take as a weight loss supplement?

There doesn't seem to be a definitive answer to that question although it seems unlikely to cause any health problems, at least if taken for short periods, but no real studies as to its safety have been undertaken [as far as I know].

The end result here is that there may be some weight loss from using Garcinia Cambogia Extract but the effects are so tiny as to be practically unnoticeable.

GLUCOMANNAN.

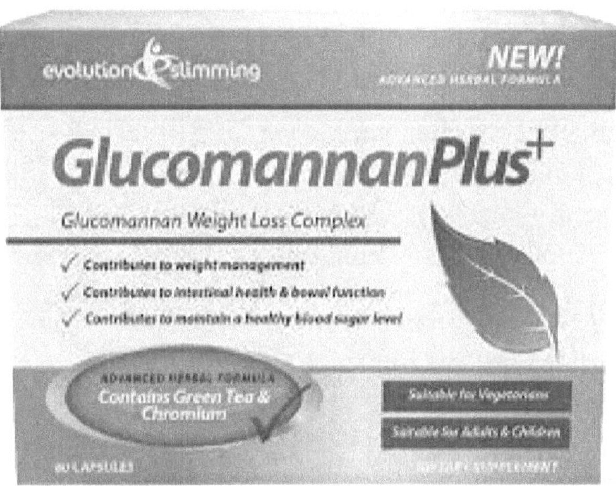

Glucomannan is a fibre found in the root of a yam.

So, what is a "yam"?

You may well ask.

Often confused with the humble sweet potato loved by so many, a yam is, in fact, a completely different plant, found primarily in Africa, Asia and Central and South America.

Grown for their tubers [roots] which is the part of the plant that is eaten, the yam is very high in fibre and it's this fibre which contains the Glucomannan used in weight loss products.

The Glucomannan sits in the gut when it's consumed and absorbs water to become like a gel in our stomach and so gives us a feeling of being "full".

When we feel full we are less inclined to over-eat and so we consume fewer calories.

Studies have shown that those who use Glucomannan in combination with a healthy diet can lose up to 5 kilos in just a few weeks; Glucomannan has also been shown to lower blood sugar, triglycerides and bad cholesterol and is very effective at relieving constipation.

On the downside, Glucomannan can cause bad wind, bloating and diarrhoea and may possibly interfere with some medications.

Overall Glucomannan seems to be a good addition in our weight loss strategy as it appears to do much more good than harm to our general health but, as always, we should consult our weight loss professionals before we use it.

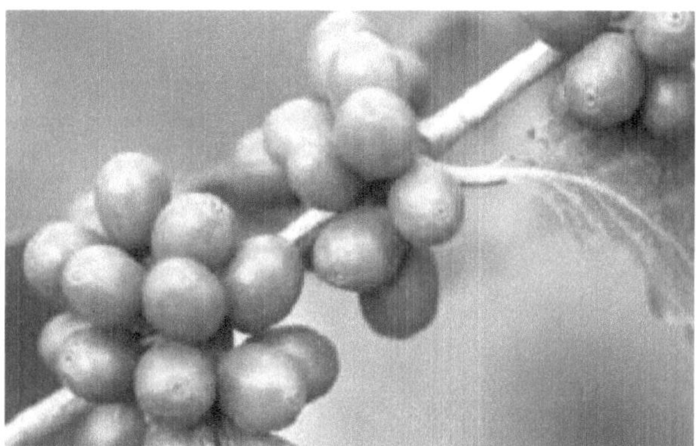

Green coffee beans are just normal coffee beans which are still as they came off the tree, they haven't been processed.

Not only do they contain caffeine but also another substance, called chlorogenic acid, which is also touted as a weight loss aid.

While the caffeine may increase the amount of fat we burn the chlorogenic acid apparently slows down the absorption of carbs in our stomach.

Again some very small studies, all industry sponsored, show that green coffee bean extract may help us with our weight loss as well as provide other health benefits such as the lowering of blood sugar levels and the reducing of blood pressure and green coffee bean extract is also high in antioxidants.

The bottom line here is that while green coffee bean extract may have some weight loss benefits it isn't scientifically proven to be effective to any measureable degree.

GREEN TEA EXTRACT.

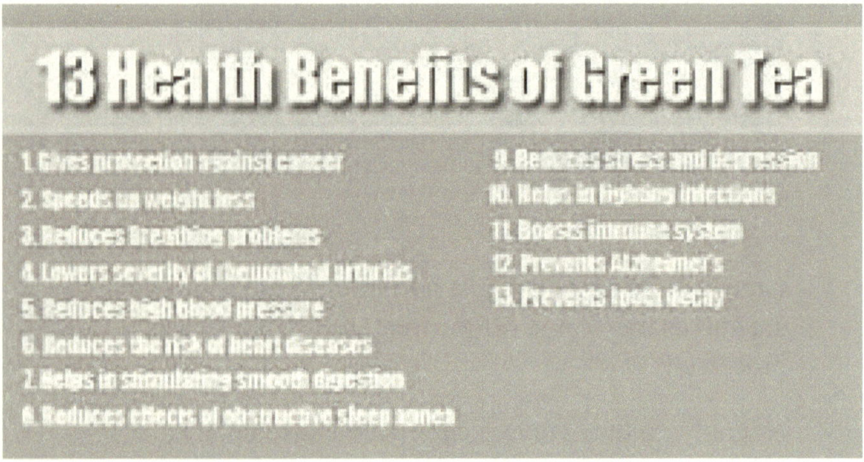

Green tea extract, as with green coffee bean extract, is high in antioxidants, the main one being epigallocatechin gallate [EGCG to the uninitiated].

As well as being a very powerful antioxidant EGCG actually has been shown to aid weight loss to some small degree, especially around the belly fat area.

Believed to increase the production of norepinephrine, a hormone which aids the body to burn fat, green tea extract is a key ingredient in many weight loss supplements and with the added benefit of its antioxidant properties green tea extract and perhaps just green tea may be a weight loss supplement worth a try just don't expect it to work miracles.

GUAR GUM.

As I've said, elsewhere and often, there is no magic formula when it comes to losing weight, a good healthy diet and sensible exercise are the only ingredients that really work in any weight loss program but many people still chase the easy fix, the "pop a pill or two and lose 10 kilos a week" solution to being overweight.

This is one of the enduring reasons the weight loss industry continues to make so much money and so little difference in the lives of those they claim to help.

We're all looking for the easy answer, the result without the work, but guess what, just as in every other area of life, it doesn't exist!

One of those products which claim to offer us an easy way out of our obesity is Guar Gum.

It's proponents claim that Guar Gum is full of soluble fibre, which is true, that it will leave us feeling fuller for longer, which is also true, and Guar Gum when added to processed food as a thickening agent is generally considered to be safe but we now find it being used as a meal replacement or a natural weight loss pill by the commercial weight loss industry and it has the potential to cause a number of digestive and intestinal problems.

Manufacturers of Guar Gum claim it can reduce our appetites by swelling and absorbing a large amount of liquid in our gut however the FDA recently disputed the efficacy of Guar Gum, especially in the product marketed as Cal-Ban 3000, as a weight loss supplement pointing out that as a weight loss product, when taken to excess Guar Gum can form very high amounts of gel in our stomach which in turn can cause obstructions in our oesophagus and intestines.

Although proven to be ineffective for weight loss, Guar Gum is still available over the counter in one form or another, it pays us to read the label carefully on any supposedly "natural" weight loss supplement to ensure that we're not taking something which has the potential to do us more harm than good.

GUARANA.

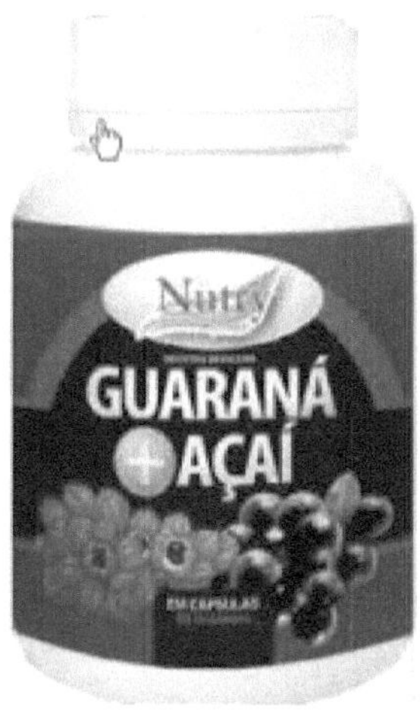

Guarana is a herb found primarily in the Amazon jungle [that's the South American jungle not the Amazon internet jungle] and it has been used quite effectively for centuries by the peoples of that region as a natural medicine.

Guarana is a stimulant and as a weight loss supplement can be quite effective as it contains twice as much, or more, caffeine than does coffee, in fact it's the richest known natural source of caffeine in the world.

We see guarana as the major ingredient in most energy drinks with the promise that it will boost energy levels, what they don't say is that the energy boost comes from the caffeine in the guarana and the energy boost it will give us is more like a very major buzz.

What does this mean for those of us on our own weight loss journey?

Guarana belongs in a class of weight loss supplements which cause thermogenesis, in effect it will boost our metabolism and therefore cause our bodies to burn fat faster than they otherwise would and it should also tend to curb our appetites.

The trick with thermogenesis is to find a product which will burn the fat without the side effects which can be very similar to those we experience when we drink too much very strong coffee.

Even if we don't experience the jitters, the nervousness or the heart palpitations when we take guarana there is no benefit to taking more of it in an effort to lose more weight more quickly, it doesn't work that way, by taking more guarana all we're doing is increasing the likelihood of us getting the side effects with no extra benefit.

It is important when we take any thermogenetic product that we increase our consumption of water to help control our body heat, that we don't be tempted to skip meals because thermogenesis may lower our blood sugar levels and that we don't take them at night or we won't sleep.

As with any stimulants guarana may increase our heart rate and blood pressure and we should be especially careful if we're taking any blood thinning medication, the best course, as always, is to talk to our doctor before we start to take any product with guarana in it.

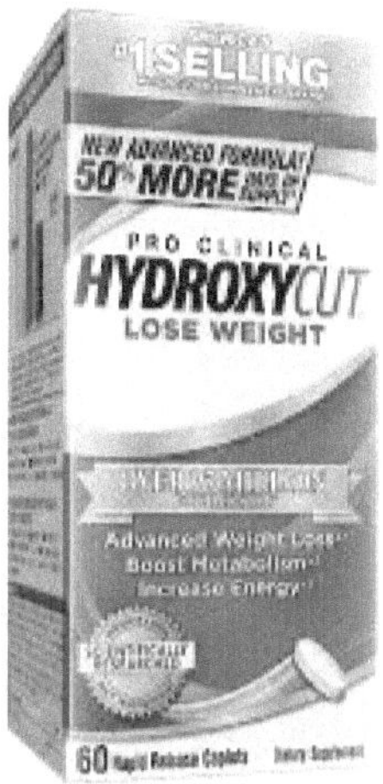

Not just one weight loss supplement but a whole suite of them, "Hydroxycut" is a family of weight loss supplements which are sold both over the counter and on the internet without a prescription.

Hydroxycut is actually a brand name and it's been available for more than ten years however, as far as I am aware there has only been one study in all that time into the effectiveness of Hydroxycut as a weight loss aid.

Containing any number of active ingredients such as caffeine, wild olive extract, wild mint extract and komijn extract, Hydroxycut is really unproven as a weight loss aid and may cause some irritating side effects in people who have a sensitivity to caffeine.

The bottom line is that there is little actual evidence to support the claim that Hydroxycut will help you to lose weight.

MERATRIM.

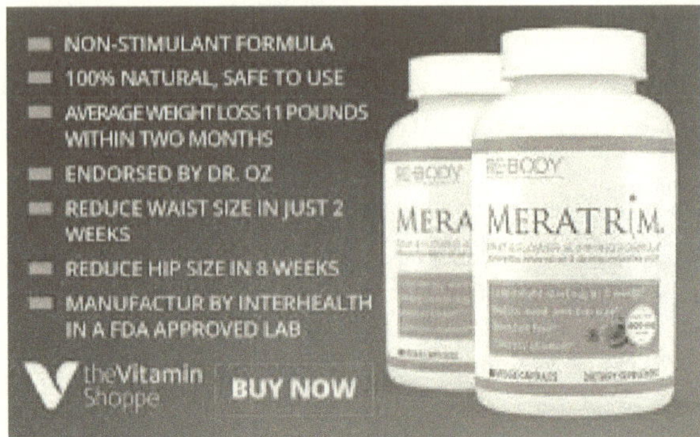

Meratrim is relatively new in the weight loss market and it's a supplement that is a blend of two plant extracts that when combined apparently make it harder for our bodies to store fat, help us to burn the stored fat we do have and reduce the multiplication of fat cells.

Sounds impressive and the results of a very limited trial seem to confirm these claims.

Of 100 obese people who took part in the trial 50 were given Meratrim, placed on a strict 2000 calorie diet and instructed to walk for 30 minutes each day while the other 50 were given a placebo and the same instructions.

The trial lasted 8 weeks and at the end of it those who took the Meratrim had lost almost twice the weight of those who took the placebo and as a bonus if you like, the Meratrim group also had other not insignificant health benefits such as reduced cholesterol, blood sugar and triglycerides.

There were also no side effects reported so it would seem Meratrim may be an answer, at least in part, to our weight loss woes but it should be noted that this was a very limited trial, it was industry sponsored and more research needs to be done before we can claim Meratrim to be our holy grail as far as weight loss is concerned

ORLISTAT [AKA ALLI].

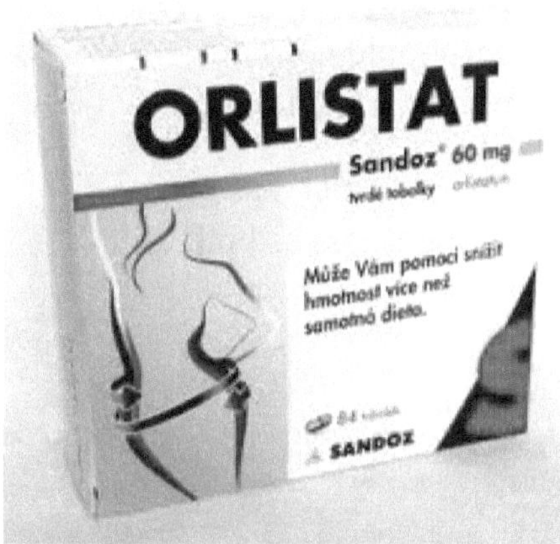

Orlistat is actually a prescription drug which you may know better as "Alli" if you purchase it over the counter or "Xenical" if you get a script for it from your physician.

Apparently inhibiting the guts ability to break down fat, Orlistat has been shown in a small number of studies to increase our weight loss by as much as 2.5 kilos when compared to a placebo.

Orlistat has also been credited with a slight reduction in blood pressure and a lesser likelihood of developing type 2 diabetes.

On the negative side, Orlistat has some quite uncomfortable side effects which may include flatulence, diarrhoea and some loss of control over bowel movements.

The fat soluble vitamins such as vitamins A, D, E and K which our bodies need may also become deficient.

If you're going to take Orlistat you should consider following a low fat diet to help reduce the side effects.

A better option may be a low carb diet which has been proven to be as effective for our weight loss as both Orlistat and a low fat diet combined.

RASPBERRY KETONES.

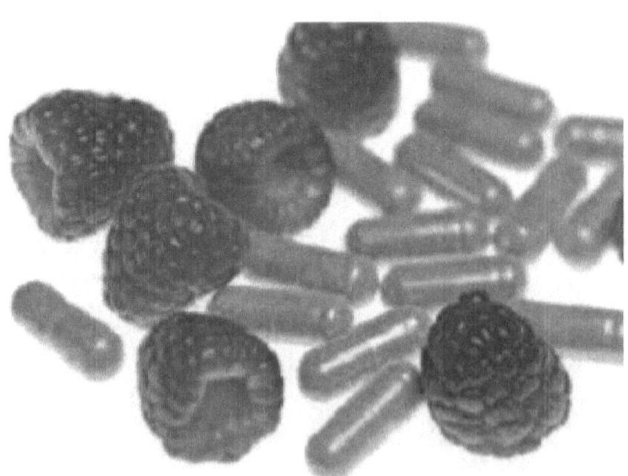

As I've quoted elsewhere on the website from the Mayo Clinic:

"For example, raspberry ketone supplements are marketed as clinically proven, natural weight-loss products.

As of November 2014, the results of only one clinical trial with raspberry ketone had been published.

The results include the following information:

"The eight-week trial used a multi-ingredient supplement with raspberry ketone, caffeine, bitter orange, ginger root extract and garlic root extract, as well as other herbs, vitamins and minerals.

Seventy obese adults were randomly assigned to receive either the supplement or an inactive ingredient (placebo).

All of the participants were placed on a restricted diet and exercise program.

Forty-five people completed all eight weeks of the trial.

Among people completing the trial, the average weight loss in the supplement group was 4.2 pounds (1.9 kilograms).

The average weight loss in the placebo group was 0.9 pounds (0.4 kilograms).

While the difference between the two groups was significant, the weight loss in the treatment group was still modest.

And the trial was only eight weeks, which is not long enough to know if the supplement will help promote weight loss over the long term.

Because the supplement included multiple ingredients, it's not possible to judge which ingredients caused a treatment effect.

Therefore, the size, method and duration of the trial provide insufficient evidence to draw conclusions about the potential benefits of raspberry ketone."

In rats, again a single study often quoted, researchers found that raspberry ketones increased the breakdown of fat and increased the levels of adiponectin, a hormone thought to be related to weight loss.

This was only one study which used massive amounts of raspberry ketones to produce, what the promoters of the product will tell you is scientific evidence that raspberry ketones will indeed aid your weight loss.

You decide!

THERMOCERIN.

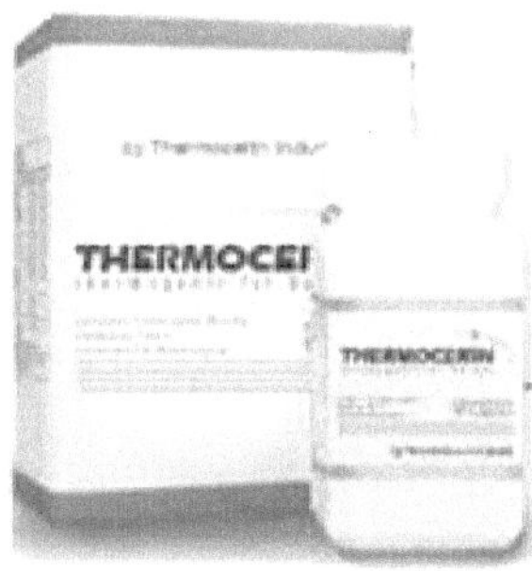

Thermocerin has as its claim to fame that it teaches our bodies to actually increase the heat they produce thereby speeding up our metabolism and as a result burning more calories and promoting weight loss.

Thermogenesis, the technical term from which Thermocerin gets its name, means, according to the Oxford Dictionary, "The production of heat, especially in a human or animal body."

So we can see how Thermocerin makes its claim to promote weight loss by heating up our bodies and so increasing our metabolism but that's not all, it also claims to search out the fat cells in our bodies and burn them off as well.

The next two questions are: What is in Thermocerin, what's its makeup and, of course, does it work?

Well Thermocerin contains a number of herbs, chemicals which occur naturally in plants such as white tea and green tea, capsaicin, which is the substance that makes chillies hot, and yohimbe which has a number of side effects and is of questionable value.

Does Thermocerin work?

There is some anecdotal evidence to suggest that it does however the jury is still out on that and it should be noted that even though it is supposedly all natural if you have an allergy to certain herbs then be wise and check with your health professional before you take it.

Last point about Thermocerin, it used to be available on prescription but that is apparently no longer the case, you can still purchase it online but be careful.

Natural diuretics, also called water pills, are a staple of the weight loss industry and for good reason, they actually work, but before you get too excited at this let's stop for a minute and try to explain why they work.

Any diuretic will cause us to lose weight, when we drink copious amounts of coffee for example, apart from getting the shakes we also find ourselves urinating more than normal.

Coffee is a natural diuretic and this is one of the effects of taking a diuretic, it makes us lose water therefore it stands to reason that the weight we then lose is water weight and we'll most likely put it straight back on when we next take a good drink of water.

This may be fine if we have a need for some very quick, short term weight loss but it doesn't work over time.

Another thing to consider is that taken independently of any other compound water pills don't really do the job nearly as effectively as when taken in conjunction with other products and when we start to mix natural diuretics with other drugs we may already be taking, for weight loss or something else, we run the not inconsiderable risk of other medical complications.

Juniper seeds can cause renal failure, equistine can cause brain damage, horsetail has been shown to cause convulsions and so on.

The bottom line here is that water pills or other natural diuretics give us the impression that we're losing weight but what we're actually losing is "water weight" and the prolonged use of these products in conjunction with other prescribed or over the counter medications can be dangerous to our health and should only be undertaken after consultation with our doctor.

PART THREE – RECIPES.

Just a few lightweight recipes for you to try, I'm sure you'll find plenty more when you look.

BREAKFAST.

VANILLA QUINOA AND ROASTED BLUEBERRY.

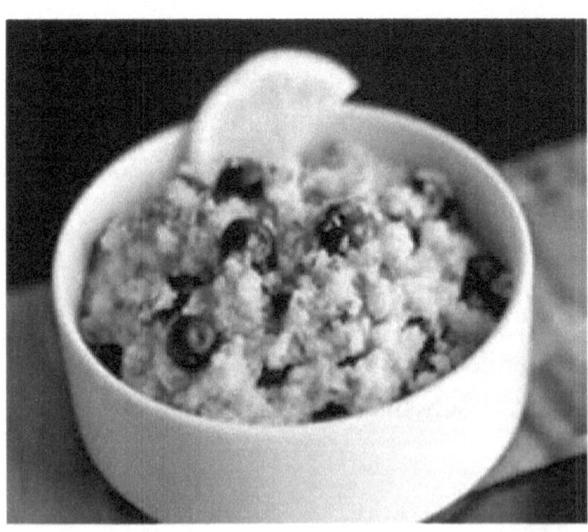

Ingredients.

1/2 cup uncooked quinoa, rinsed and drained

1 1/4 cups Silk Light Vanilla Soymilk

Pinch of salt

2 teaspoons agave nectar

1 teaspoon vanilla extract

1/2 pint fresh blueberries

1 teaspoon agave nectar

2 tablespoons toasted unsweetened coconut

2 tablespoons toasted sliced almonds

Method:

Preheat oven to 450 degrees.

Line a baking sheet with foil and spread the blueberries out in a single layer.

Toss the blueberries in a teaspoon of agave nectar until they are coated.

Place the blueberries on the middle rack of the oven and roast them for 8-10 minutes or until they have released some of their juices but are still holding their shape.

While the blueberries are roasting, bring the quinoa, vanilla soymilk, and pinch of salt to a boil in a small saucepan.

When the quinoa comes to a boil, turn the heat down to low, cover the saucepan with a lid, and let the quinoa simmer for 15-20 minutes or until all of the soymilk is absorbed.

Remove the cooked quinoa from the heat and stir in 2 teaspoons of agave nectar and 1 teaspoon of vanilla extract.

Pour the quinoa into two bowls and top with the roasted blueberries, coconut, and sliced almonds.

BREAKFAST YOGURT PARFAIT.

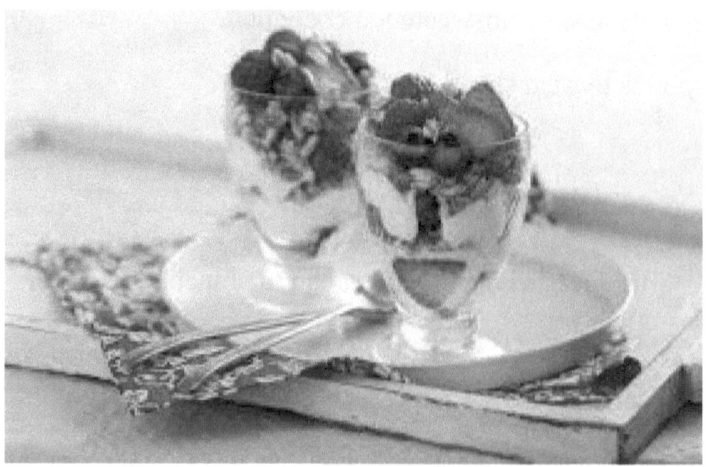

Whether you eat this at home or on the go, this recipe delivers protein and fruit in a breakfast that's less than 190 calories.

Ingredients.

3 cups vanilla nonfat yogurt

1 cup fresh or defrosted frozen strawberries in juice

---

1 pint fresh blackberries, raspberries or blueberries

1 cup good quality granola

Method.

Layer 1/3 cup vanilla yogurt into the bottom each of 4 tall glasses.

Combine defrosted strawberries and juice with fresh berries.

Alternate layers of fruit and granola with yogurt until glasses are filled to the top.

Serve parfaits immediately to keep granola crunchy.

AVOCADO BREAKFAST PIZZA.

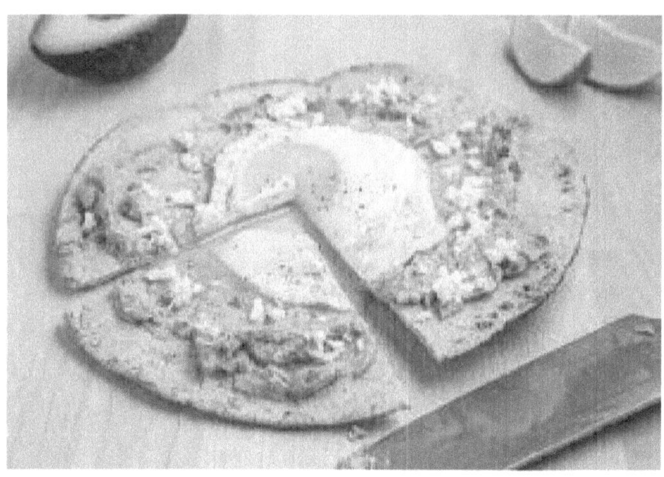

This weight loss recipe is easy to make. It has just 252 calories per serving, and it's packed with superfoods like egg and avocado.

Ingredients.

Pizza Dough

6 slices crispy bacon

2 avocados

Fresh lime juice

Salt & pepper

Cayenne (red) pepper (optional)

Arugula

2 scallions, sliced thin

Method.

Make your pizza dough or pick up a disc at your local pizza place or market.

Preheat oven to 400 degrees.

Shape into 1 large pizza or 3 small ones.

Lightly flour your baking or pizza pan, place the shaped dough onto it. With your fingertips, lightly oil the top of the dough with grapeseed or olive oil. Season with salt & pepper.

Bake for 15-18 minutes or until dough is golden (8-10 minutes for smaller pies).

While the dough bakes, mash your avocados, add in about a tablespoon of lime juice as well as a good amount of salt & pepper. Taste and adjust. If you like a little heat, add in some Cayenne pepper or minced jalapeno.

Once the dough is finished baking, spread the mashed avocado on top, sprinkle with arugula, bacon and scallions.

Cook 3 eggs on your stove top and place them on-top of the pie(s).

You can also choose to use flatbread for the pizza if you choose.

SWEET POTATO PANCAKES.

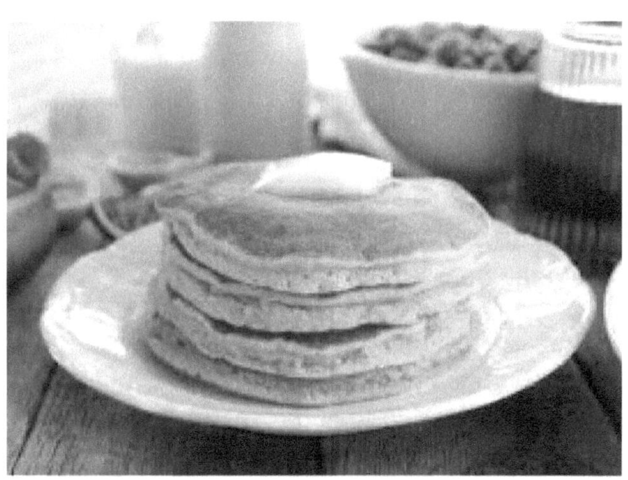

Ingredients.

3/4 pound sweet potatoes

1 1/2 cups all-purpose flour

3 1/2 teaspoons baking powder

1 teaspoon salt

1/2 teaspoon ground nutmeg

2 eggs, beaten

1 1/2 cups milk

1/4 cup butter, melted

Method.

Place sweet potatoes in a medium saucepan of boiling water, and cook until tender but firm, about 15 minutes. Drain, and immediately immerse in cold water to loosen skins. Drain, remove skins, chop, and mash.

In a medium bowl, sift together flour, baking powder, salt, and nutmeg. Mix mashed sweet potatoes, eggs, milk and butter in a separate medium bowl. Blend sweet potato mixture into the flour mixture to form a batter.

Preheat a lightly greased griddle over medium-high heat. Drop batter mixture onto the prepared griddle by heaping tablespoonfuls, and cook until golden brown, turning once with a spatula when the surface begins to bubble.

SLOW COOKER CREAMY ALMOND OATMEAL.

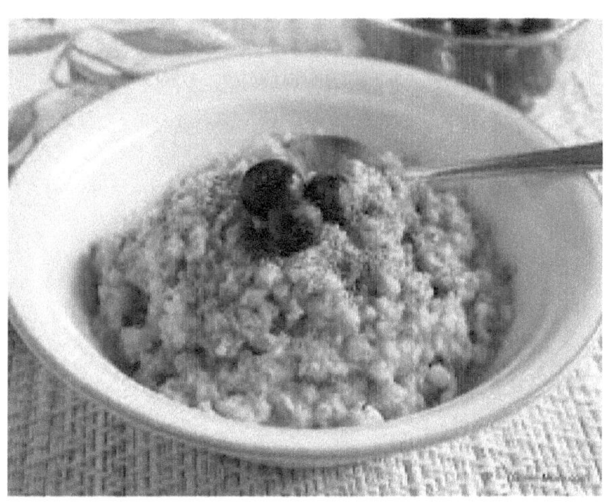

Ingredients.

1/2 cup steel cut oats

2 cups almond milk, unsweetened

3 tablespoons honey or maple syrup

Pinch sea salt

1/2 teaspoon cinnamon

2 tablespoons diced almonds

Method.

Combine in slow cooker the oats, almond milk, honey, salt, and cinnamon. Whisk ingredients until well combined.

Cover and cook on low for 4-5 hours, or until desired consistency. Sprinkles almonds on top and serve.

With steel-cut oats, this is one of those recipes for weight loss that will fill you up in all the right ways. It delivers an itty-bitty 129 calories in each serving!

SLOW COOKER FRENCH TOAST CASSEROLE.

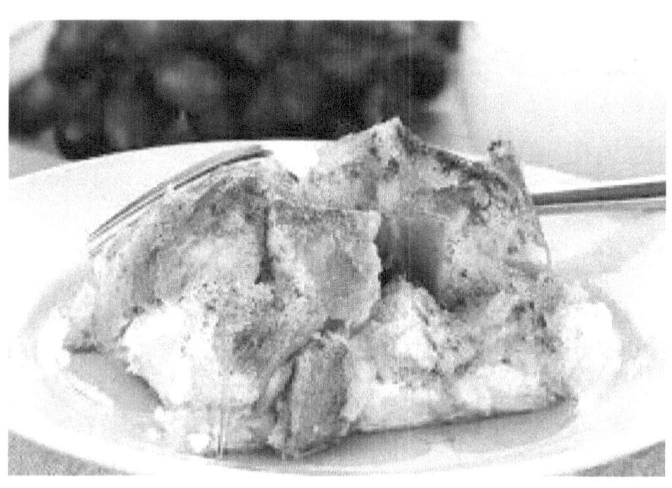

Ingredients.

---

1 loaf of bread sliced or diced Recipe for Homemade French Bread

6 eggs

2 cups milk (Dairy Free Alternative can be used)

1/2 tsp cinnamon

Topping.

1/4 cup butter (or Dairy Free Margarine) Softened

1/2 cup firmly packed brown sugar

1 tsp cinnamon

1/2 cup chopped pecans

Dash of nutmeg

Method.

Whisk together eggs, milk and cinnamon and pour over diced bread in a large bowl. Cover and let it soak overnight in the fridge or at least 4 hours.

When ready to bake spray the inside of the crockpot (4-6 quart sized works best) to avoid sticking. Pour in Bread Mix.

In a small bowl mix together butter, brown sugar cinnamon, pecans and nutmeg.

Crumble of the top of the bread mix. Cover and Cook on low for 4 hours...or if you are in a hurry High for 2 hours.

Let sit for 15-20 minutes and serve!

PITA POCKET BREAKFAST SANDWICH.

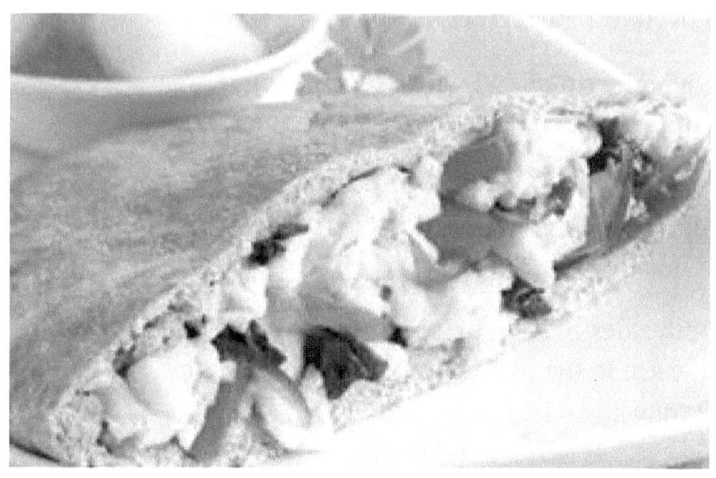

Ingredients.

2 large eggs

2 large egg whites

1 tablespoon milk

1 cup baby spinach torn into small pieces

4 grape tomatoes sliced in half lengthwise

2 green onions, diced

Sea salt and pepper to taste

¼ cup Feta cheese crumbles

1 whole wheat pita pocket, cut in half

2 teaspoons olive oil

Method.

Preheat oven to 350 degrees.

In a medium mixing bowl whisk together eggs, egg whites, milk, spinach, tomatoes, green onions, and salt and pepper to taste.

Pour egg mixture into an 8" non-stick skillet, place in oven on middle rack.

Brush both sides of each pita half with olive oil, place on foil and warm in the oven during the last 2 minutes of cooking time.

Cook eggs approximately 15 to 18 minutes or until puffy and just set in the centre, but not hard. Sprinkle on the feta cheese and return to the oven for one more minute.

Remove skillet from oven, cut omelette in half and place each half in a pita pocket. Press edges into warm pita and serve immediately.

BIG 5 SUPERFOOD SMOOTHIE.

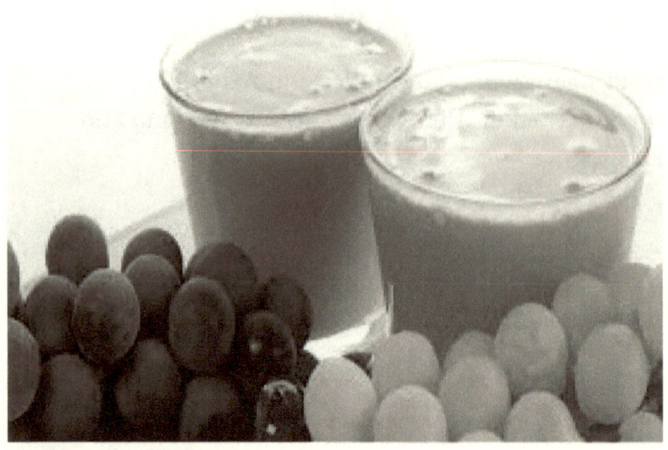

Ingredients.

1 organic (sweet) apple, cored, keep peeling

1 cup frozen red grapes

1 teaspoon freshly grated ginger

1/2 cup kefir, plain, fat free

1/2 cup chilled green tea, unsweetened, home brewed is best

1 tablespoon honey (optional)

ice cubes

Method.

Add all the ingredients to a blender and blend until smooth. Add amount of ice according to thickness preferred.

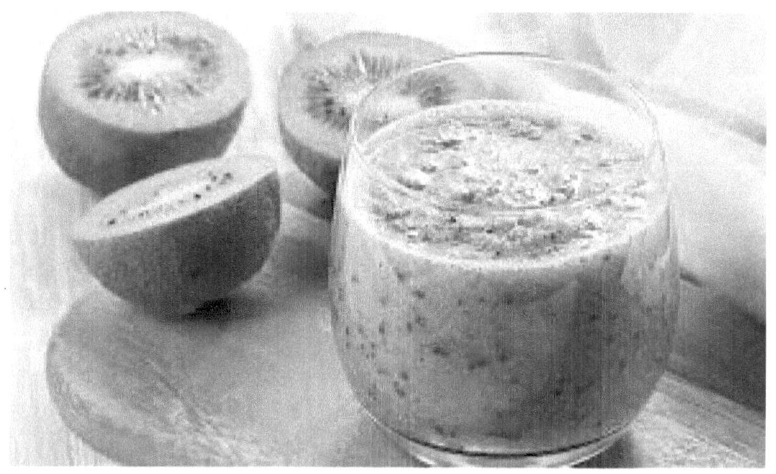

Ingredients.

1 banana

4 strawberries

1 kiwi fruit, peeled

2 cups kale (organic), loosely packed

1-1/2 cups green tea (home brewed...no sweeteners added)

6 ice cubes

Add all the ingredients to a blender and blend until smooth. Add amount of ice according to thickness preferred.

POMEGRANATE BANANA GINGER BLAST.

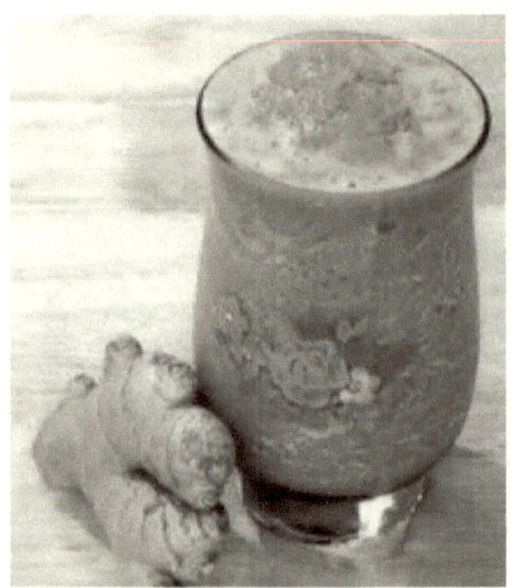

Ingredients.

1 frozen banana, pre-slice before freezing

1/2 cup plain Greek yogurt, fat-free

Ginger Root, 1/4 "of knuckle (knuckle = length of finger joint)

1 cup pure pomegranate juice, no added sugar

4-5 ice cubes

Method.

Blend all ingredients until smooth.

ROASTED PEAR SANDWICH WITH BABY SPINACH.

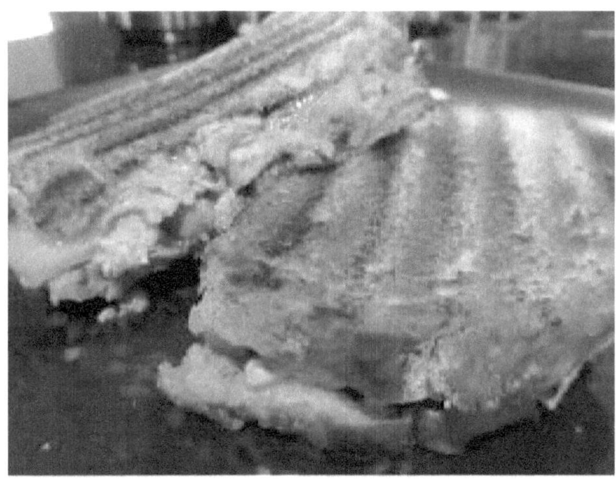

Ingredients.

2 Pears of medium firmness, peeled, cored and seeded

2 teaspoons canola oil

1 teaspoon freshly squeezed lemon juice

1 cup baby spinach

4 slices whole grain artisan bread, cut bread horizontally

Method.

Preheat oven to 400 degrees.

Combine canola oil and lemon juice in a medium bowl.

Cut pears into ½" slices and gently toss in oil and lemon juice.

Place pears on rimmed cookie sheet and roast 20 minutes, or until pears are tender and lightly golden.

Toast bread and add favourite condiment or goat cheese yogurt spread to one side of each slice, top with spinach and pears, lightly press bread together.

GARDEN SALAD WITH LEMON PEPPER VINAIGRETTE

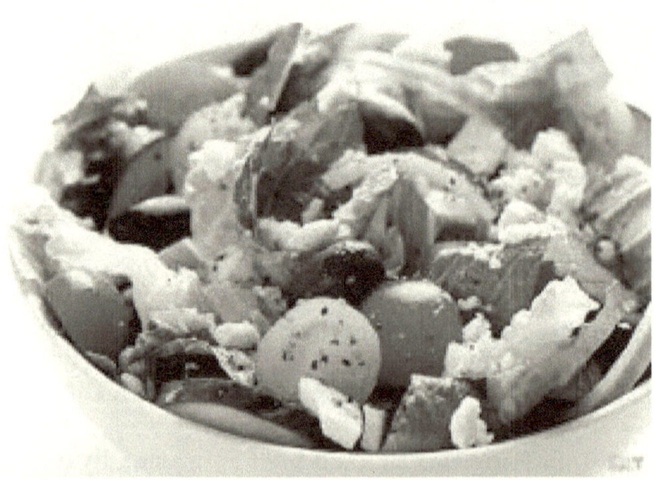

Ingredients.

1/4 cup olive oil

2 tablespoons vinegar

1 tablespoon McCormick Perfect Pinch Lemon & Pepper
Seasoning

1 tablespoon sugar

Garden salad.

2 heads leaf lettuce, rinsed and torn into bite-size pieces

1 package (8 ounces) mushrooms, sliced

1/2 red onion, thinly sliced

10 cherry tomatoes, halved

1/2 avocado,

10 thin slices of cucumber,

A little spinach

SEAFOOD CHOWDER.

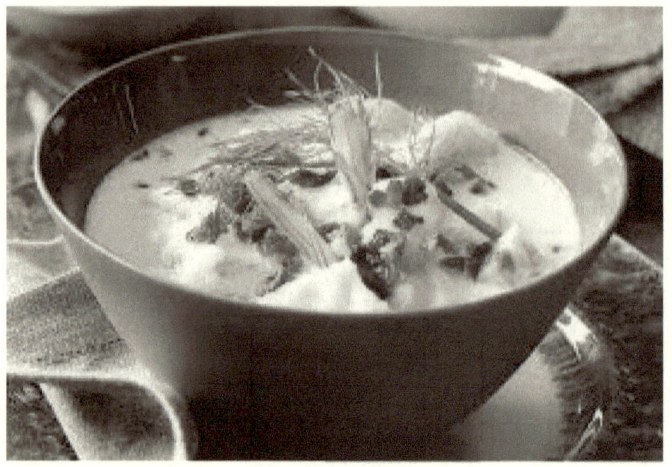

Ingredients.

400g firm white fish, cut into large chunks

1 leek, washed and sliced

2 cloves garlic, crushed

3 short cut bacon slices, diced

3 tsp. cornflour mixed with ¼ cup cold water

3 large potatoes, diced

1/2 cup corn

2 cups skim milk

2 cups fish stock

2 tbsp. olive oil

Squeeze juice 1 lemon

Cracked pepper

Method.

In a large pot heat ½ oil and cook bacon for 4mins. Add remaining oil and leeks, turn down heat to med and sauté leeks for 5-8 mins. Add garlic and cook for 1 minute longer.

Place your potatoes and corn into pot with stock and milk, turn heat down to low and simmer for 10 mins or until potatoes are nearly cooked.

Season with cracked pepper.

Now add the fish and lemon juice, and simmer for 5 minutes.

Thicken sauce with cornflour and water mixture, should thicken in 1 minute, and continue to stir.

Serve immediately with a slice of crusty bread and garnish with chives.

LOW CAL CHICKEN SALAD.

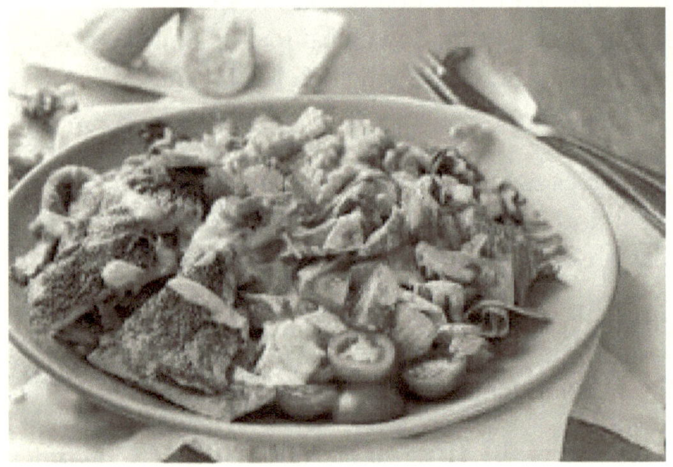

In a large bowl, combine:

Two diced cooked chicken breasts

1 cup thin sliced celery

1 cup seedless red grapes

2 Tbsp finely diced red onion

1/2 cup plain Greek yoghurt

1 tsp Dijon mustard

1 splash hot sauce, such as Tabasco – optional

Method.

Combine gently, cover, & chill for an hour or two in the refrigerator.

Serve on butter lettuce leaves

VEGGIE & PESTO SANDWICH.

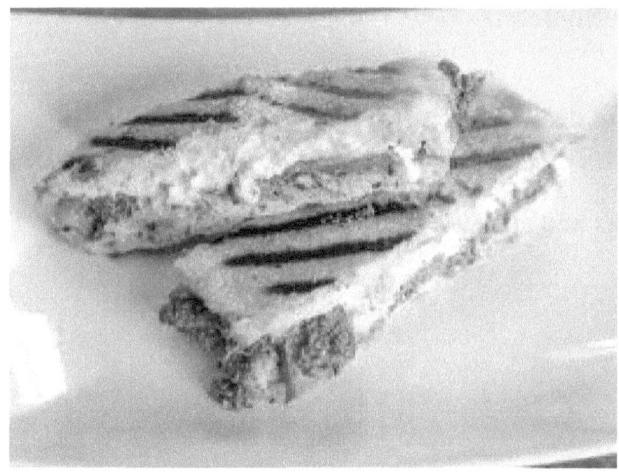

Ingredients.

1 small eggplant, thinly sliced

2 zucchini, thinly sliced

2 Tbsps olive oil

4 rolls (hamburger buns, Kaiser or French)

3 cup homemade or prepared pesto

2 tomatoes, sliced

1 avocado, sliced

1 box alfalfa sprouts

Salt and pepper

Method.

Heat a stove top grill or heavy skillet over high heat.

Lightly brush eggplant and zucchini with oil and grill 3
to 4 minutes, turning once, until vegetables are blackened
a bit around edges.

Spread rolls with pesto and layer on grilled vegetables,
tomatoes and avocado.

Top with sprouts and sprinkle with salt and pepper to
taste.

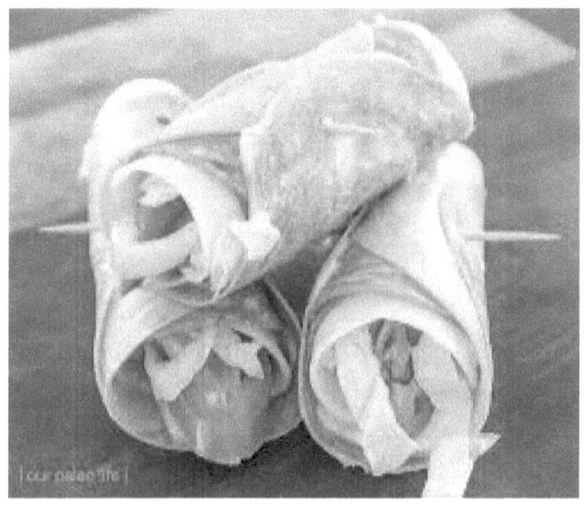

<u>Avocado Dressing.</u>

[Enough for 2 servings Turkey Roll-Ups]

Ingredients.

1/3 cup paleo sour cream

1 ripe avocado, peeled and diced

Juice of one lime

1/2 tsp of chilli powder

1/2 teaspoon ground cumin

2 garlic cloves, finely chopped

1 scallion, chopped

Pinch of salt

1/2 cup chopped cilantro leaves, plus more for garnish

Method.

Place dressing ingredients in blender and blend until smooth and creamy.

Paleo Turkey Roll-Ups

Yield: Serves 2

Ingredients.

4 slices turkey

4 pieces romaine lettuce

2 tomato slices, cut into four pieces

4 slices cucumber, cut in half

2 slices bacon, cooked and crumbled

Method.

Place one slice of turkey on a cutting board.

Put lettuce, tomato, cucumber, bacon crumbles and a dollop of dressing on top of turkey.

KALE CAESAR SALAD.

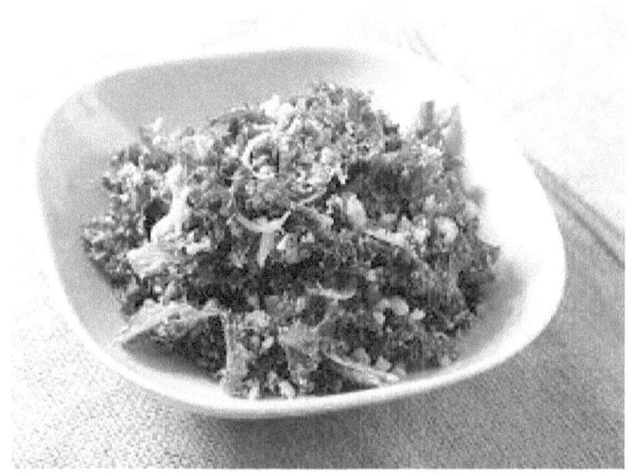

Ingredients.

Extra virgin olive oil

4 cloves garlic, smashed

Pinch of crushed red pepper

2 slices of day-old Italian bread, cut into 1/2-inch cubes

1/2 cup grated Parmesan cheese

Zest and juice of 1 lemon

1 tablespoon Dijon mustard

2 to 3 anchovy fillets

2 shakes Worcestershire sauce

Salt

1 bunch of kale, tough stems removed, cut into ribbons

Method.

Coat a large saute pan with olive oil.

Toss in half the garlic and the crushed red pepper and bring the pan to medium heat.

Cook the garlic until it becomes golden and very aromatic, 2 to 3 minutes.

Remove the garlic and ditch it-it is now surplus to requirements.

Toss in the bread cubes and cook, stirring frequently, until they are golden, crisp, and have absorbed all the oil.

Remove from the heat and place to one side.

In the bowl of a food processor, combine the Parmesan cheese, lemon zest and juice, the remaining garlic, the Dijon, anchovies, and Worcestershire. Puree until the mixture is smooth, 15 to 20 seconds.

With the machine running, add 1/4 to 1/3 cup olive oil through the feed tube.

Let the processor continue to run for another 10 to 15 seconds.

Taste and season with salt if needed.

In a large bowl, toss the kale with the croutons and two-thirds of the dressing.

Let the kale sit for 3 to 4 minutes to soften.

Taste, add the remaining dressing, and adjust the seasoning if needed.

CHICKEN NOODLE SOUP.

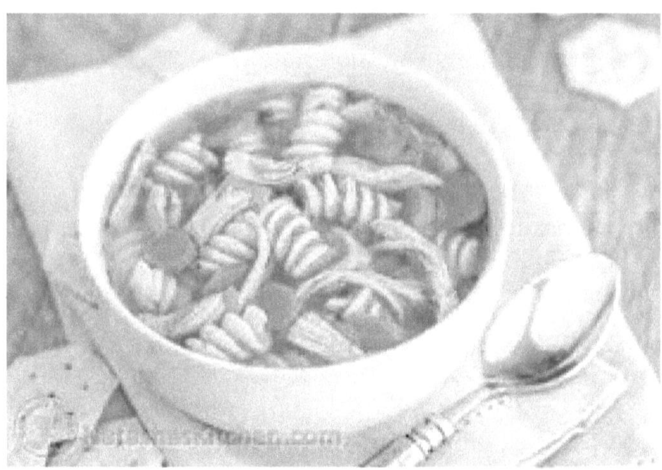

Ingredients.

20g butter

1/2 cup (85g) chopped onion

1/2 cup (85g) chopped celery

2 litres liquid chicken stock

2 cups (500ml) liquid vegetable stock

250g chopped cooked chicken breast

1 1/2 cups (200g) egg noodles

1 cup (140g) sliced carrots

1/2 teaspoon dried basil

1/2 teaspoon dried oregano

Salt and pepper to taste

Method.

In a large pot over medium heat, melt butter.

Cook onion and celery in butter until just tender,

Pour in chicken and vegetable stocks and stir in chicken, noodles, carrots, basil, oregano, salt and pepper.

Bring to a boil, then reduce heat and simmer 20 minutes.

GRILLED CHICKEN AND BLUEBERRY SALAD.

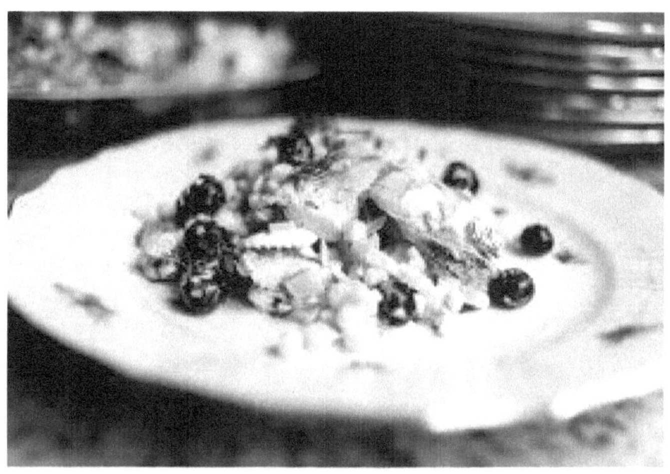

Ingredients.

5 cups mixed greens

1 cup blueberries

¼ cup slivered almonds

2 cups cubed chicken breasts, cooked

Dressing.

¼ cup olive oil

¼ cup apple cider vinegar

¼ cup blueberries

2 Tbsp honey

Salt and pepper to taste

Method.

In a large bowl, toss the greens, blueberries, almonds,
and chicken breasts until well mixed.

For the salad dressing, combine the olive oil, apple cider vinegar, blueberries, and honey in a blender. Blend until smooth.

Add salt and pepper to taste.

PANZANELLA AND ROCKET SALAD.

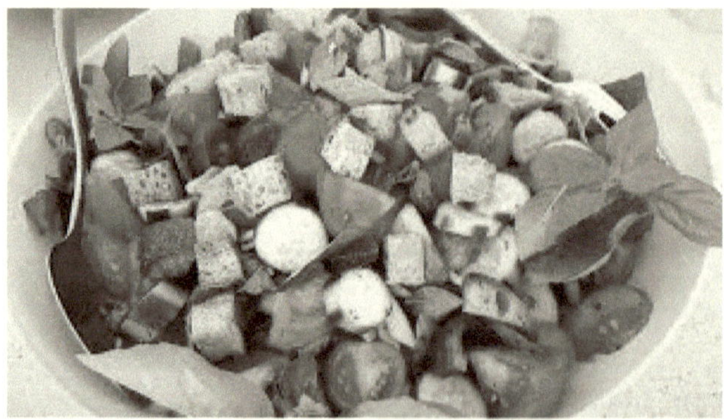

Ingredients.

1 large garlic clove, minced

1/2 cup extra-virgin olive oil

1 ciabatta loaf, cut into 2.5cm cubes (12 cups)

1/4 cup red wine vinegar

1 teaspoon salt

1/2 teaspoon freshly ground black pepper

500g assorted heirloom tomatoes, cut into 1.5cm cubes

500g fresh mozzarella cheese cut into 1cm cubes

3/4 cup chopped fresh basil

1/2 cup baby rocket

1/4 cup finely chopped shallots

Method.

Prepare the barbecue for medium-high heat.

Using a large heavy knife, mash the garlic with a pinch of salt into a paste.

Transfer the garlic to a small bowl and add 1/2 cup of olive oil in a slow stream, whisking until combined well.

Brush the bread slices with 1/4 cup of the garlic oil. Grill until golden, about 5 minutes per side. Cut the bread into cubes.

Whisk the vinegar into the remaining garlic oil.

Season the vinaigrette to taste with salt and pepper.

In a large bowl, toss the grilled bread, tomatoes, mozzarella, basil, rocket, and shallots with enough vinaigrette to coat.

Let stand 10 to 15 minutes at room temperature to allow the flavors to develop, then toss again just before serving.

DINNER.

MEDITERRANEAN STUFFED CHICKEN BREAST.

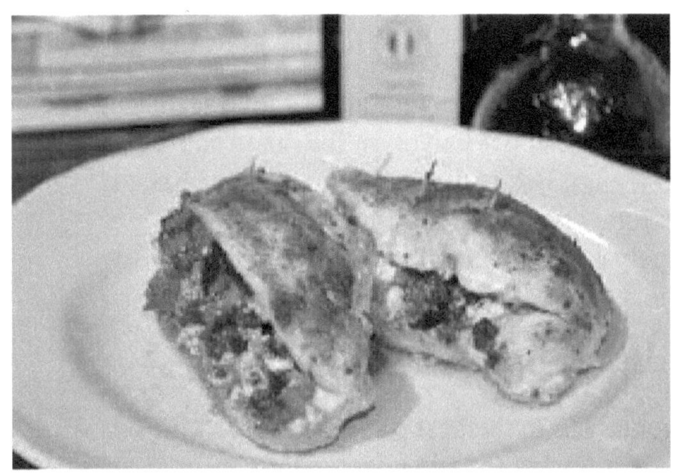

Ingredients.

1 red bell pepper

2 garlic cloves, minced

1/4 cup feta cheese, crumbled (1 ounce)

2 tablespoons olives, finely chopped

1 1/2 tablespoons fresh basil, minced

1/4 teaspoon salt

1/4 teaspoon black pepper

8 boneless skinless chicken breasts

Salt and pepper, to taste

Dried basil, to taste

Method.

Preheat broiler.

Cut bell pepper in half lengthwise and remove seeds and membranes. Place pepper halves on foil-lined baking sheet, skin side up. Broil 15 minutes or until blackened. Place in air-tight container for 15 minutes. After 15 minutes, finely chop the 2 bell pepper halves.

Mix together chopped bell pepper, garlic, cheese, olives, basil, salt, and pepper in a bowl.

Cut a horizontal slit in thickest portions of each chicken breast to form a pocket (but do not cut all the way through). Spoon the pepper/feta/olive mixture into each pocket. Close the opening with a toothpick. Season chicken on both sides with salt and pepper, and sprinkle the top side with dried basil.

Place chicken on broiler rack, and broil 6-8 minutes each side, or until done (it may take additional time, depending on thickness of the chicken breasts). Remove from oven, loosely wrap with foil and let stand 10 minutes before serving.

HERBED SALMON WITH BROCCOLI RISOTTO.

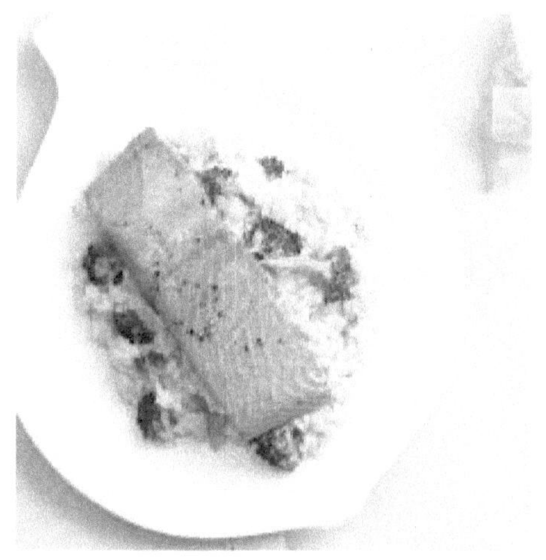

Ingredients.

Salmon:

1 lb. skin-on salmon fillet

Salt

Freshly ground black pepper

Broccoli

1.5-2 c. small broccoli florets

½ tsp. salt

Toasted Orzo:

1 Tb. unsalted butter

1 Tb. olive oil

1 small onion, chopped

2 cloves garlic, minced

1 cup dry orzo

2¼ c. chicken or vegetable stock

½ tsp. kosher salt

¼ tsp. freshly ground black pepper

Juice & zest of one 1 lemon

Handful fresh parsley, chopped

¼ c. freshly grated parmesan

Method.

Prepare Salmon:

Heat oven to 350 degrees.

In a non-stick, oven-proof pan, sprinkle a little olive oil and heat to medium/high.

Sprinkle fish with a little salt and pepper.

Place fish in warm pan, skin side down, so it starts to sear.

After a few minutes, turn off heat and place pan in oven to allow the fish to finish cooking -- this takes about 10-15 minutes, depending on thickness of your fillet. Cook until the flesh flakes apart, then remove from oven and allow to rest a bit. Remove skin and dark areas at the skin line. Break up the fillet into small pieces; set aside until ready to use.

Prepare Broccoli:

While salmon cooks, bring a saucepan of water and ½ tsp. salt to boil. Drop in broccoli pieces and blanche about 5 minutes. Remove with a slotted spoon and place broccoli in ice water for a few minutes. Transfer to a bowl and set aside until ready to use.

Prepare Toasted Orzo:

In a non-stick pan, add butter and olive oil and heat to medium.

Add chopped onion and garlic and mix until coated. Cook to slightly translucent (about 5 minutes).

In a separate pan, simmer the stock and keep over low heat until ready to use.

Add orzo to the onion mixture and stir to combine. Stir frequently as the orzo browns over medium heat (about 5-7 minutes).

Reduce heat to medium/low, then add about ½ c. of warm stock to the orzo mixture and allow it to slowly be absorbed by the orzo (reduce heat if it's bubbling too rapidly). Before it gets too dry, add another ¼ - ½ c. of stock, stir well, and allow it to be slowly absorbed. Keep doing this until all the liquid is fully absorbed and the orzo is tender.

Add salt and pepper, along with lemon juice, zest and parmesan. Mix well.

Add salmon and broccoli, then sprinkle with a little more lemon juice and parsley just before serving.

SLOW COOKER CHICKEN CHILLI.

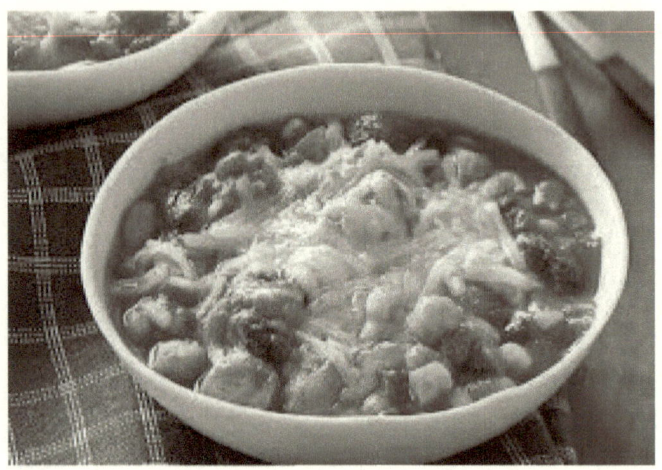

Ingredients.

1 teaspoon vegetable oil

2 skinless, boneless chicken breast halves

2 cups chicken broth

1 (15 ounce) can black beans, rinsed and drained

1 (15 ounce) can cannellini beans, drained and rinsed

1 (14.5 ounce) can diced tomatoes, drained and rinsed

1/2 yellow onion, chopped

1 1/2 tablespoons chili powder, or more to taste

---

1 clove garlic, minced

1/2 teaspoon ground cumin

1/2 teaspoon paprika

1/2 teaspoon mustard powder

1/2 teaspoon garlic powder

1 dash hot sauce (such as Cholula®), or to taste

1 pinch salt and ground black pepper to taste

1/2 cup sour cream or Greek yoghurt.

Method.

Lightly grease the crock of your slow cooker with vegetable oil.

Put chicken breasts into the bottom of the slow cooker crock; add chicken broth, black beans, cannellini beans, diced tomatoes, yellow onion, chili powder, garlic, cumin, paprika, garlic powder, hot sauce, salt, and black pepper.

Cook on Low for 6 hours (or on High for 3 hours).

Remove chicken breasts from the crock to a cutting board. Shred chicken into strands with a pair of forks and return it to the mixture in the crock; add sour cream and stir.

Continue cooking on Low for 30 minutes more.

SLOW COOKER ROPA VIEJA [CUBAN BEEF].

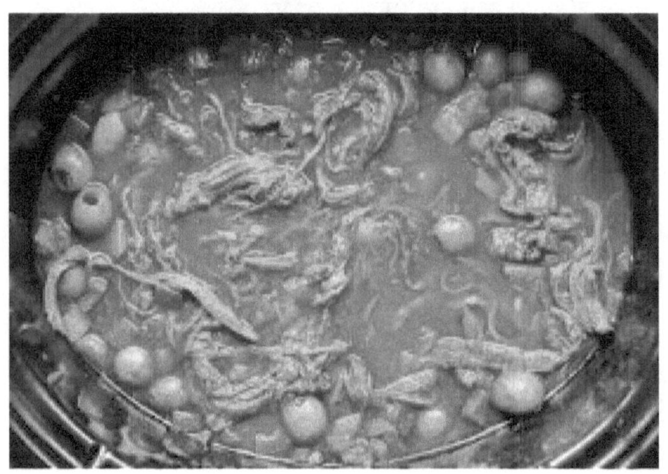

Ingredients.

3 lbs. beef flank steak

1 cup beef broth

1 (6-oz.) can tomato paste

1 (14-oz.) can petite diced tomatoes

1.5 tsp. salt

¼ tsp. pepper

---

1 tsp. oregano

1 tsp. cumin

½ tsp. turmeric

1 Tbsp. apple cider vinegar

1 small white onion diced

2 bell peppers, diced

1 cup Spanish olives

3 whole garlic cloves, peeled

Cooked yellow rice for serving

Slow Cooker Size: 4-quart or larger

Add the beef broth, tomato paste, diced tomatoes, salt, pepper, oregano, cumin, turmeric and apple cider vinegar to the slow cooker. Stir.

Add the flank steak and flip it around in the sauce so it gets coated. Add the bell pepper, onion, olives and garlic cloves, mix those items together to combine on top of the meat.

Cover and cook on low for 9 hours on LOW without opening the lid during the cooking time. Shred the meat with 2 forks right in the slow cooker.

SLOW COOKER BEEF CURRY.

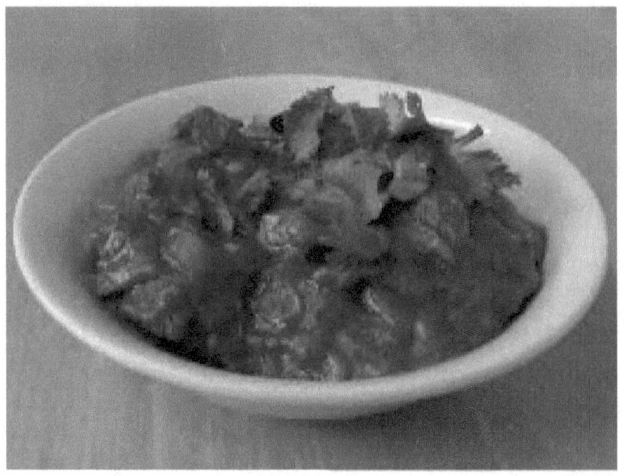

Ingredients.

2 1/2 pounds cubed beef stew meat

1 pound small red-skinned potatoes, quartered

2 tablespoons Madras curry powder

1 1/4 teaspoons ground cumin

2 tablespoons finely chopped peeled ginger

2 large cloves garlic, grated

Salt and freshly ground pepper

5 slices naan bread

2 15-ounce cans diced fire-roasted tomatoes

1 1/4 cups fresh cilantro

1/4 cup sliced pickled jalapeno peppers, plus 1
tablespoon brine from the jar

Method.

Toss the beef and potatoes with the curry powder, 1
teaspoon cumin, 1 tablespoon ginger, the garlic, 1
teaspoon salt and a few grinds of pepper in a 6-quart
slow cooker.

Crumble 1/2 slice of naan into small pieces over the beef
and potatoes, then pour in the tomatoes.

Cover and cook on low, 7 hours.

Uncover and skim off any fat from the top of the mixture.

Stir well to combine, then let stand 10 minutes.

Meanwhile, combine the cilantro, pickled jalapenos and
brine, 1/4 cup water and the remaining 1/4 teaspoon
cumin and 1 tablespoon ginger in a food processor.

Pulse until combined; season with salt and pepper.

Stir 3 tablespoons of the cilantro puree into the slow
cooker; season with salt and pepper.

Reserve 2 cups beef curry for Beef and Vegetable
Handpies.

Serve the remaining curry with the naan; top with the
remaining cilantro puree.

SLOW COOKER SIZZLING CHICKEN FAJITAS.

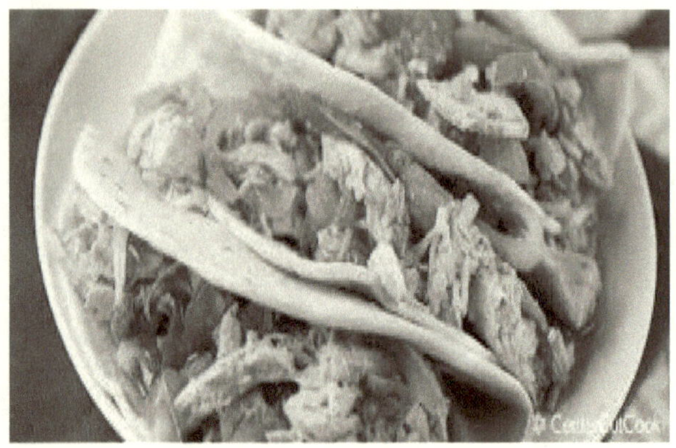

Ingredients.

4 boneless, skinless chicken breasts

3 bell peppers, sliced

1 onion, sliced

1 packet taco seasoning

3 tablespoons lime juice

Fixings:

Tortillas

Cheese

Sour cream

Shredded lettuce

Beans

Rice

Guacamole

Salsa

Method.

Arrange the onions and peppers on the bottom of a slow cooker

Place chicken on top of the veggies

Sprinkle taco seasoning and lime juice over everything

Cook on low for 8 hours or high for 4 hours

Using two forks, shred the chicken

Return chicken to slow cooker and combine with vegetables and juices. Stir to mix well

Dish and serve hot with fixings

JUICY "NOT FRIED" CHICKEN.

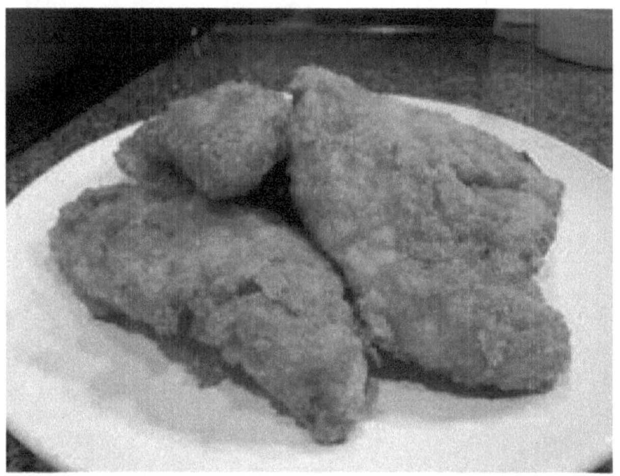

Ingredients:

1/2 cup non-fat buttermilk, OR 1/2 tablespoon lemon juice(or vinegar) mixed with (1/2 cup) 1 percent milk

1-1/2 tablespoons Dijon mustard

2 cloves garlic, minced

2 teaspoons hot sauce

6 medium to large (2 to 2 1/2 pounds) chicken breasts (not boneless), skin removed

1/2 cup white whole-wheat flour

1 1/2 teaspoons paprika

1 teaspoon dried thyme

1 teaspoon baking powder

1/8 teaspoon salt

Freshly ground black pepper to taste

Method.

Preheat oven to 425 degrees F [220 degrees C]

In a wide and shallow bowl, whisk together the buttermilk, mustard, garlic, and hot sauce.

Add chicken and flip to coat on both sides.

Line a baking sheet with parchment paper.

Whisk the flour, paprika, thyme, baking powder, salt and pepper in a small bowl.

Place the seasoned flour in a bowl with an airtight lid. Add the chicken 2 pieces at a time and shake with the lid on. Remove the chicken, shake off any excess flour, and place it on the parchment lined baking sheet..

Coat the top and sides of the chicken with cooking spray or brush with olive oil. Bake the chicken until golden brown and no longer pink in the center, 40 to 50 minutes.

ZESTY ASIAN CHICKEN MEATBALLS.

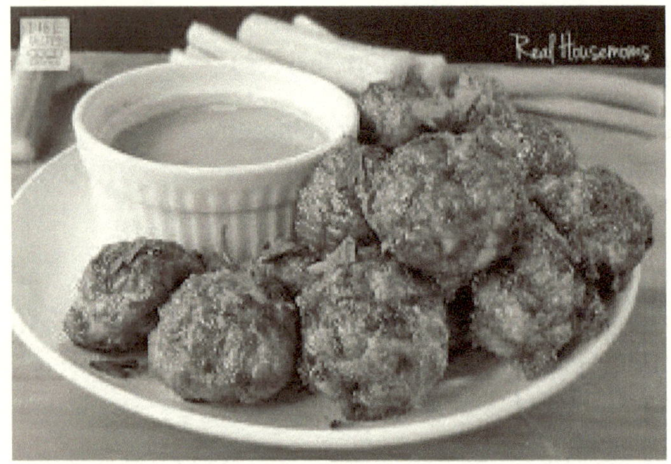

Ingredients

Meatballs:

1 3/4 – 2 lbs. ground chicken (or turkey)

6 scallions, chopped (whites + greens)

5 garlic cloves, minced (or grated)

1 inch piece of ginger, grated

1 tablespoon Chinese five spice powder

1/2 tablespoon sea salt

2 large egg, room temperature

1 cup breadcrumbs

2 tablespoons low sodium soy sauce

1 1/2 tablespoons sesame oil

For the hoisin glaze:

1/2 cup hoisin sauce

1/4 cup low sodium soy sauce

2 teaspoons sambal oelek (optional)

2 tablespoons rice vinegar

1/2 teaspoon ginger powder (see note)

1/4 cup brown sugar

Method.

Position 2 racks near the center of the oven and preheat to 475°F [250°C]

Line to baking sheets with parchment paper, set aside.

In a large bowl, combine the ground chicken, scallions, garlic, ginger, five spice, salt, eggs, panko, soy sauce, and sesame oil. Use your hands to mix all the ingredients together. It's easier to tell when the ingredients are combined when using hands. Do not over mix, it will result is drier meatballs.

Shape the meat mixture into balls, about 3 tablespoons of meat per ball. You could also do this with an ice cream scoop. Place shaped meatballs on prepared baking sheet. Bake for 11-13 minutes or until the meatballs are completely cooked.

While meatballs are baking prepare the sauce. Combine all the ingredients for the sauce in a small saucepan and bring to a boil over medium heat. Reduce the sauce by 1/4, about 3-4 minutes once the sauce boil. When the sauce has thicken remove from heat.

Using 2 tablespoons, dip each individual meatball into the sauce. Alternately, you can brush each meatball with the sauce. Place back on the baking sheet and bake for an additional 2 minutes. Sprinkle with additional scallions and sesame seeds. Serve warm.

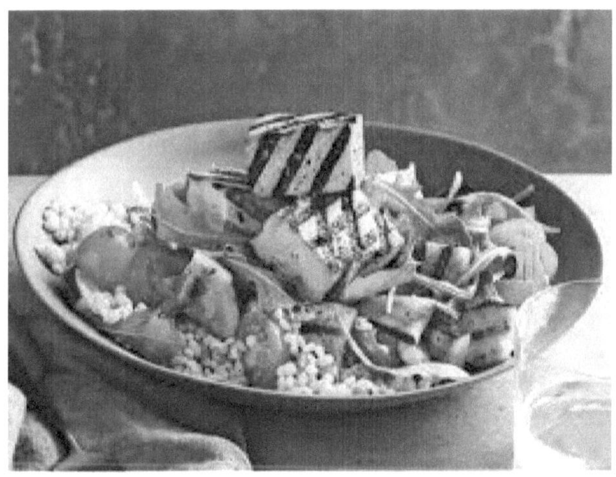

Ingredients.

Tofu:

1 pound firm tofu, frozen and thawed

3 tablespoons lite soy sauce, optional gluten-free Tamari

2 tablespoons toasted sesame oil

2 tablespoons apple cider vinegar

1 clove garlic, minced

1 teaspoon freshly grated ginger

1/4 teaspoon red pepper flakes

Vegetables:

1 tablespoon toasted sesame oil

1 pound fresh green beans, trimmed

1 red bell pepper, sliced

1 small red onion, sliced

1 teaspoon lite soy sauce, optional gluten-free Tamari

2 tablespoons Szechuan sauce

1 teaspoon corn starch

Method.

Tofu:

Once the tofu is thawed, cut it into 1/2 inch thick slices; squares or triangles will work. Combine the marinade ingredients in a small bowl. Lay the tofu in a shallow baking dish and pour the marinade overtop. Refrigerate for 30 minutes, or up to 24 hours.

Preheat your grill to medium high heat. Grill the tofu about 5 minutes per side, until firm. It should have nice grill marks on both sides.

Vegetables:

Bring a pot of salted water to a boil and add the green beans.

Blanche for 2 minutes; drain and rinse with ice cold water.

Combine the corn starch with a teaspoon of cold water. Heat a large skillet or wok over medium high heat. Add the sesame oil, followed by the green beans, red peppers and onions. Add the soy sauce (optional Tamari) and Szechuan sauce and stir quickly for about 1 minute. Add the corn starch mixture and stir until thickened.

Serve the tofu with the veggies.

ARTICHOKE AND SPINACH PASTA CASSEROLE.

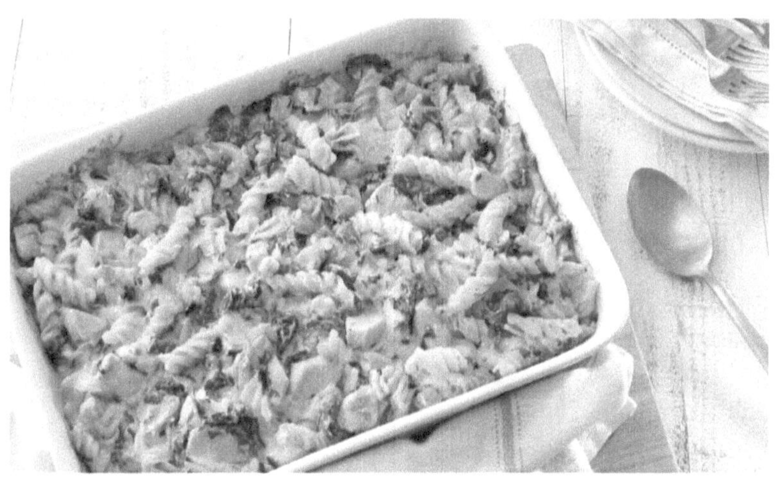

Ingredients.

2 cups (measured uncooked) cooked high fiber pasta

4 oz softened light cream cheese

¼ cup light sour cream

¼ cup reduced calorie mayo

---

2 garlic cloves, diced

4 cups fresh chopped spinach

6oz can artichoke hearts (drained)

⅓ cup light shredded mozzarella

1 Tbsp finely grated parmesan cheese

Dash of salt & pepper

Method.

Preheat oven to 350F, spray a 9x13 casserole dish with some cooking spray

In a bowl mix together your cream cheese, sour cream, mayo, artichoke, spinach, garlic, salt & pepper and mozzarella.

Toss in your cooked drained pasta and mix well.

Spread out into your casserole dish, sprinkle parmesan cheese on top and bake in oven for approx 25 minutes.

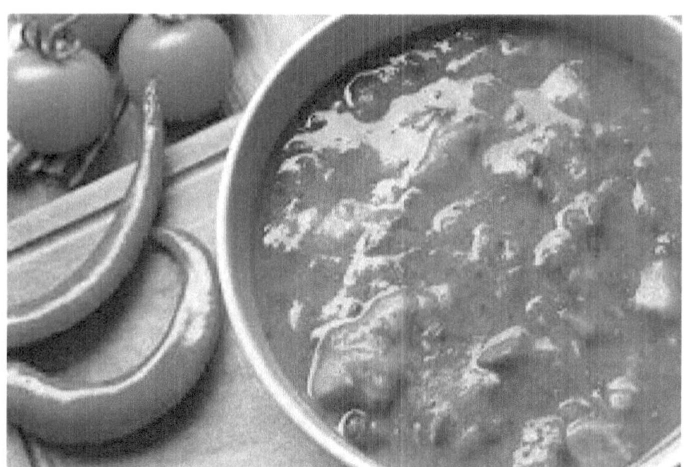

Ingredients.

1 1 lb lean ground turkey

1 large onion, diced

1 green bell pepper, diced

---

1 (4-ounce) can diced green chillies

2 cloves garlic, finely minced

2 tablespoons chilli powder

2 teaspoons ground cumin

½ teaspoon cinnamon

1 (32-ounce) package chicken stock, reserve ¼ cup

2 (14.5-ounce) cans cannellini or great northern beans, drained and rinsed, divided

2 (15-ounce) cans diced fire roasted tomatoes

¼ cup wine

1 cup shredded Cheddar cheese

Method.

Cook ground turkey as specified on the package. Always cook to well-done, 165°F as measured by a meat thermometer. Add onion, bell pepper, chilies, garlic, chili powder, cumin and cinnamon; stir. Turn heat to high and continue to cook 5 minutes or until veggies begin to caramelize.

Add chicken stock, one can of beans, tomatoes and wine. Stir to combine. Reduce heat to medium. Cover to simmer. In food processor (or blender) add one can beans, Cheddar cheese and reserved ¼ cup chicken stock. Process mixture until smooth. Add pureed bean mixture to stock pot and stir to incorporate. Remove from heat and let stand 5 minutes to thicken.

DESSERTS.

BERRY PARFAIT.

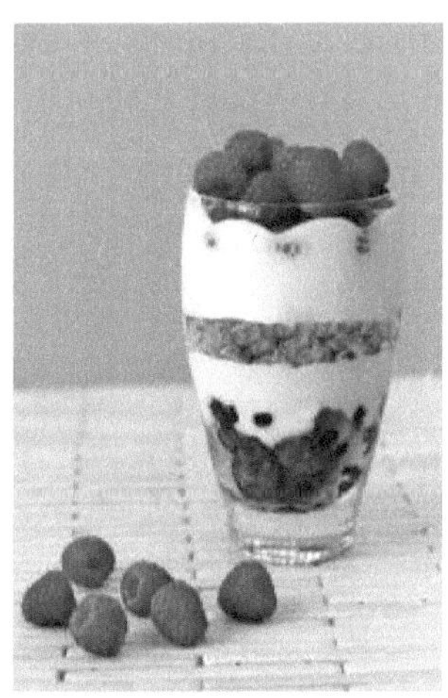

Ingredients:

1 1/2 cups fresh raspberries

2 cups fresh blueberries

1 cup ricotta cheese

8 oz plain Greek yogurt

1 tbsp raw honey

3 tbsp granulated stevia

1 tbsp fresh lemon juice

1 tbsp lemon zest

1 tsp vanilla extract

Method.

Blend all ingredients (except berries) in a large mixing bowl until well combined

Starting with the raspberries, layer the berries with the filling ending with the blueberries on top in a tall parfait glass.

Chill for a few hours and serve.

MINI BANANA PUDDING.

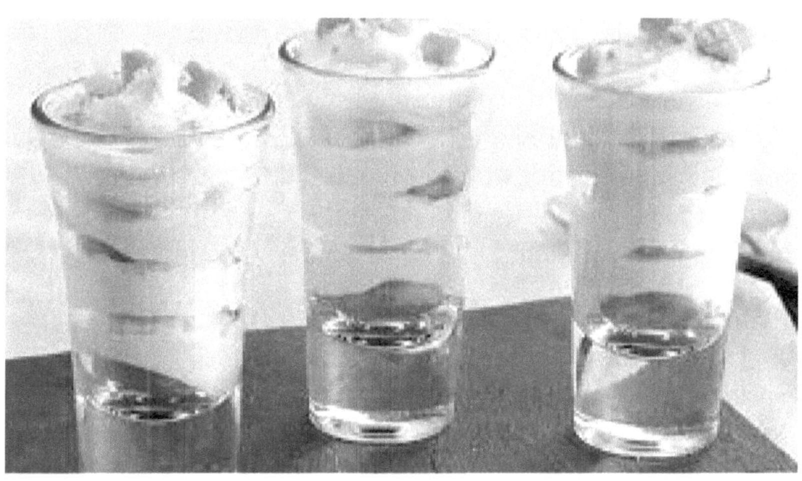

Ingredients.

10 whole almonds

2 tablespoons cornstarch

Dash of sea salt

3 tablespoons coconut palm sugar

1 egg yolk, slightly beaten

3/4 cup milk or canned lite coconut milk

1/2 teaspoon vanilla

2 bananas, thinly sliced

6 (4 ounce) dessert dishes

Method.

Preheat oven to 325 degrees f. Roast almonds 12 minutes and allow to cool while preparing pudding. After cooled, mince almonds in a food processor or use a knife.

In a saucepan, combine cornstarch, salt and sugar. Add egg yolk to dry ingredients. Gradually stir in milk and continue stirring until well combined. Turn to medium heat and cook while stirring constantly. Continue cooking until a pudding like consistency.

Remove from heat, stir in vanilla. While still warm, alternate pudding with bananas in dessert dishes. Sprinkle minced almonds on top of pudding. Top with whipped topping if desired.

MINI BLUEBERRY CHEESECAKE.

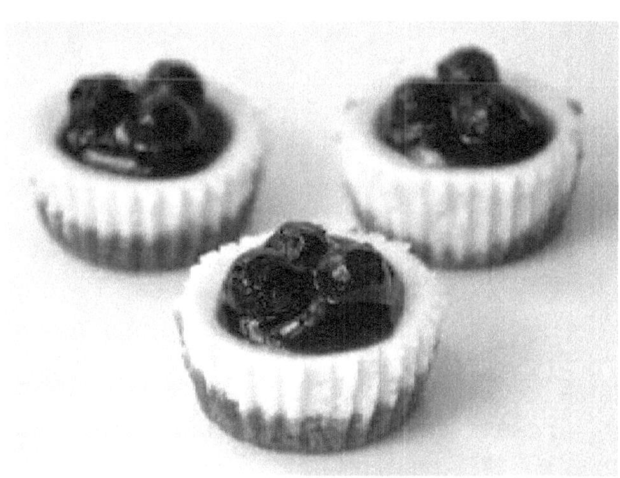

Ingredients.

Crust:

6 oz Sugar-free Shortbread cookies

2 Tbsp. applesauce

Cheesecake filling:

2 8oz. ⅓ less fat cream cheese

2 Tbsp. non fat (or low fat) Greek yogurt

1 tsp. vanilla extract

1 Tbsp. skim milk

1 egg

1 Tbsp. cornstarch

3 Tbsp. sugar

Topping:

3 cups of chopped fresh blueberries

2 Tbsp. honey

Method.

Crust:

Pulse cookies in the blender or food processor to get fine crumbs. In a small bowl, mix the cookie crumbs with applesauce until all combined. Line a 12-cup muffin pan with foil cupcake liners (just the foil part). Gently press some of the cookie crust mixture on the bottom of each cup, covering the bottom and a little bit up the sides.

(You would use roughly ½ Tbsp of mixture for each cup.)

Preheat the oven to 325.

Cheesecake: Beat cream cheese on medium speed until light and fluffy (about a minute). Add milk, yogurt, vanilla extract and egg, beating until mixed after each addition. Add sugar and cornstarch and mix well.

Divide the cheesecake mixture among the prepared cups, filling them to almost full.

Bake for 18 minutes then turn off the oven and open the oven door about half way (however much it will allow you but not all the way.) Let the cheesecakes sit in there for about 10 minutes.

Meanwhile, combine chopped blueberries and honey on a small sauce pot, over medium-low heat. Stir well, cover and let them cook until soft and tender (about 15 minutes). Stir the blueberries occasionally. Take off heat and set side when they are done.

Top cheesecakes with some blueberries topping as you serve them. This cheesecake can be served warm or cold!

MINI QUINOA ALMOND JOY BARS.

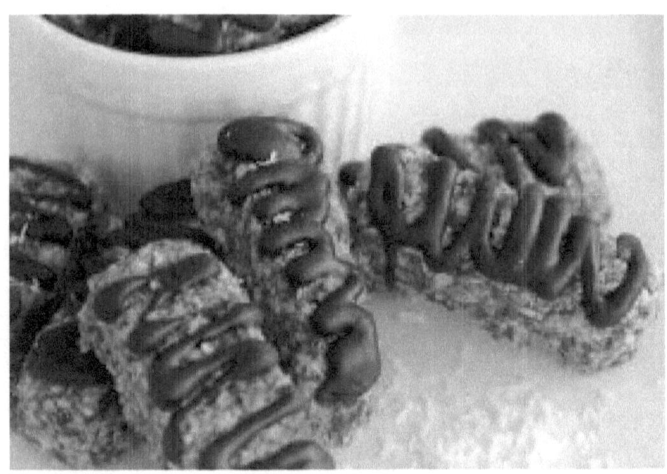

Ingredients.

1/3 cup (dry) quinoa

2/3 cup water

12 whole dates, no sugar added

1/2 cup whole almonds with skins (optional 1/2 coarse almond meal)

1/2 cup finely grated coconut

2 - 3 teaspoons water

1/4 cup semi-sweet chocolate chips, (for gluten-free chips we used Enjoy LIfe)

Method.

Add quinoa and water to a small saucepan, cover and bring to a boil, reduce heat to a simmer and cook approximately 15 minutes or until all water has been absorbed. Cool to room temperature and refrigerate at least 2 hours...overnight will work. One cup cooked quinoa can be used if already made.

Add dates, almonds, coconut, and cooked quinoa to the food processor and pulse until ingredients are well combined and a ball forms. Return ingredients to the mixing bowl, and add one teaspoon of water at a time, until mixture holds together. Shape into 14 - mini bars.

In a small saucepan, add chocolate chips and melt over low-heat or in a double-boiler. Drizzle warm chocolate over each bar. Refrigerator and allow chocolate to harden. Bars can be stored in an airtight container for several days or frozen in a freezer safe dish.